The LOTUS KITCHEN

Happy Yoga &
Good Eating

Much Love,

Gwen
Kenneally

Skip

The Lotus Kitchen
Everyday Vegetarian Recipes to Nourish Yoga Practice and Inspire Mindful Eating

Skip Jennings and Gwen Kenneally

ISBN: 978-0-9906966-2-9

First published in 2015 by Huqua Press
An operating division of Morling Manor Corporation
Los Angeles, CA

Illustrated by Yoko Matsuoko
Graphic Design: Dave Shulman / designSimple
Photography: Chloe Moore

The Lotus Kitchen assumes no responsibility for any injuries sustained as a result of your yoga practice. The American Yoga Association does not recommend Yoga exercise for pregnant or nursing women or for children under 16 years of age. If you are elderly or have any chronic or recurring conditions such as high blood pressure, neck or back pain, arthritis, heart disease, and so on, seek your physician's advice before practicing.

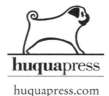

huquapress
huquapress.com

The LOTUS KITCHEN

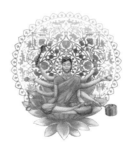

Everyday Vegetarian Recipes to Nourish
Yoga Practice & Inspire Mindful Eating

SKIP JENNINGS AND GWEN KENNEALLY

Table of Contents

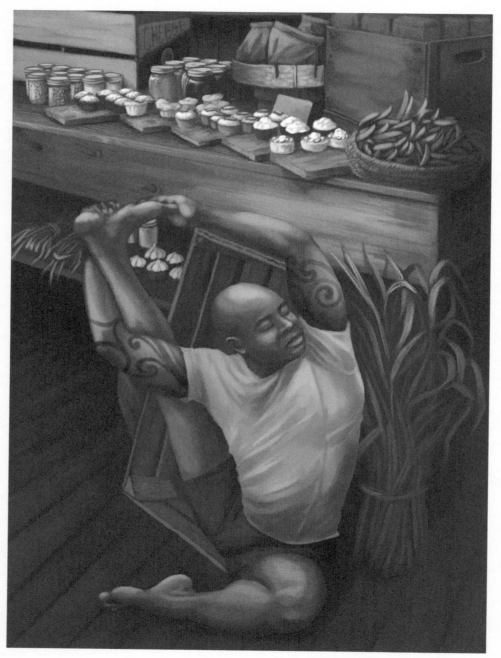

SUN DIAL (*PARIVRTTA SURYA YANTRASANA*)
This is a level three pose that focuses on lateral flexibility
while challenging balance in a seated position.

Foreword

From the ancient rishis of India, the Essenes of Palestine, to today's indigenous societies and spiritual traditions throughout the world, we find mutual agreement on how the food we eat is rich in spiritual meaning and connects us to the Divine. Is this simply a religious notion, or is there a genuine link between the nourishment food provides the body temple and what it contributes to awakened awareness? Whether it's the allegorical story about the apple tree in the Garden of Eden or the Bodhi fig tree in Bodh Gaya, it's a fascinating fact that they are connected to holy events, giving rise to the question: Is there a sacredness waiting to be discovered in something as seemingly simple as food?

If you were to research the role of food in our society, you would see that it is referred to as "fuel." The human body is not a machine; it is a temple of the living spirit within us and food is a dynamic life force that nourishes it. Donald Morse, a physician and professor at Temple University, conducted a research experiment with his students wherein they meditated for five minutes before eating. The results? The participants produced 22% more of an enzyme in saliva called alpha-amylase, which breaks down carbohydrates and B vitamins in food. The point is that when our meal ritual goes beyond filling up an empty stomach, we absorb physical, mental, and spiritual nutrients.

The wisdom in *The Lotus Kitchen* awakens our awareness to the fact that it's time we reclaim our spiritual connection to food — from how it is grown, cultivated, selected, and prepared, to the personal rituals in which we engage before, during, and after eating.

I have known Gwen Kenneally and Skip Jennings for a number of years, both as students in my classes at the Agape International Spiritual Center and as individuals who are following their hearts by delivering their gifts, talents, and skills in the world. What they have created in this book is an exquisite offering of recipes, meditations, and yoga postures that restore the sacred relationship between body and spirit. By practicing them, we can develop an entirely new relationship with food, one that evokes mindfulness, and that affirms life. This book will cause a sacred shift in your relationship with food, because as you savor your food, you will savor your life in a deep, profound way.

Michael Bernard Beckwith
Founder, Agape International Spiritual Center
Author of *Life Visioning*

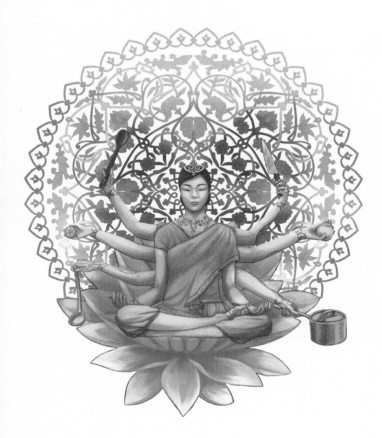

Introduction

Welcome to *The Lotus Kitchen*, a place of being and a space of the mind where yoga and vegetarian cooking entwine. This book intends to offer more than a gingerly curated collection of healthy and boldly flavored recipes; it's a culinary beacon that shines light toward an awakened way of life. It's a journey that encourages you to explore an engaged and meaningful pathway to empowerment through yoga, and to enhance your existing practice with thoughtful food preparation and mindful eating.

Furthermore, *The Lotus Kitchen* is an invitation to feed the mind, body and spirit each meal, every day, with meaning and purpose. Many of the recipes are connected to a yoga practice or meditation to support a holistic approach to being and healing. In some of the recipes we emphasize the healing properties of a given ingredient. We encourage you to contemplate food and the specific ways it nourishes and invigorates the body temple.

The notion of this book was birthed during a lively discussion about food and yoga. The vision was there and it was a matter of bringing together favorite recipes, creating new ones and preparing them over and over again until they were invited to this volume. Ours is a perfect yin-yang relationship. Gwen, a celebrated chef and daily yoga participant, made the ideal partner for Skip, a creative vegan cook, yoga instructor and fitness coach.

The word yoga means union or to yoke, bringing together two or more things. This book is a living practice of yoga, pairing the two worlds of food and yoga to inspire healthy living. This co-creation is designed to combine vegetarian cooking for the everyday cooking enthusiast with yoga practices for anyone with a reasonable familiarity with basic movements and breath work.

The Lotus Kitchen sets the intention that everyone can spend and enjoy time in the kitchen and practice yoga. We hope you will find your joy doing both. Activate the fun factor while you cook. Have patience with your dishes and never give up. If a given recipe doesn't turn out the way you planned, we ask that instead of harping on flaws you choose to see the perfection in trying a new dish.

The joy begins with choosing the recipe, and it continues through the moment you taste the first bite. Feel free to add or remove ingredients depending on your likes and dislikes. Eating is a journey that must be embraced with enthusiasm, even though our tastes for food and yoga may vary.

Yoga's history is a story of evolution. *The Lotus Kitchen* is anchored in authentic yoga principles:

• *Hatha Yoga is physical activity and prepares the body for meditation.*
• *Meditation Yoga is the practice of mindfulness that focuses on our oneness.*
• *Mantra Yoga is the spoken words that anchor the Yoga Consciousness with tonality and affirmations.*
• *Service Yoga offers the intention to bless and serve the planet.*

The Lotus Kitchen philosophy is the practice of all these types of yoga. The names and poses themselves have evolved during the past six hundred years. Some have remained the same, while others have taken on the characteristics of the region where they were first introduced. It can even shift from studio to studio, instructor to instructor. Yoga is a consciousness that anchors the physical work we do. Not every yoga pose is the right pose for each person. Keep in mind that, above all, the practice of yoga is about finding your own path to enlightenment.

The Lotus Kitchen is also the practice of being aware of what you are cooking, what you are eating, and how the body is moving. With every breath, every morsel of food, every ingredient, we invite you to be aware and awaken to the process. One of the most powerful practices of mindfulness is meditation. Meditation is simply awareness. Some spiritual avatars believe that meditation is the practice of focusing your thinking to quiet the chatter in the mind. Throughout this book we give you the opportunity to begin or increase your personal practice of meditation. It doesn't matter how long you meditate; what does matter is the intention to center your thinking and "quiet the monkey mind."

The Lotus Kitchen encourages eating from the earth. When possible we shop our neighborhood farmer's markets to procure the farm-fresh produce. Not only do we support food grown from the state and the region we live in, we know the power of using region-specific seasonal foods. Also, be flexible with what is available in your region. If you can't find a certain ingredient, feel free to substitute and experiment. Release your fears around cooking and live adventurously.

Above all, *The Lotus Kitchen* invites you to honor yourself. If there is something that disagrees with your authentic self, feel free to change the recipe or practice so it best serves you. You can take your time, and ease into the practice of cooking, mindful eating and yoga. You don't become a master overnight. Remember, it is the practice of the journey, not the destination. Be kind to yourself; practice without judgments. Your spirit is perfect and complete. Namaste.

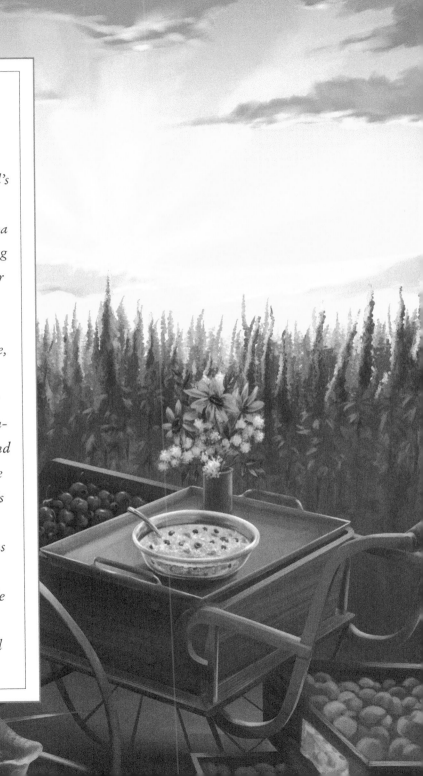

Quinoa

Quinoa is a delicately flavored grain that was a staple in the ancient Inca diet. One of the world's true superfoods, quinoa is a complete protein, containing all nine essential amino acids. Quinoa is also a great source of fiber and iron, containing more than twice as much of both than any other grain. It is the mother lode for vegetarians and vegans who are concerned about getting sufficient protein in their diets. It also contains lysine, essential for tissue growth and repair.

Although we think of quinoa as a chewy or nutty grain (similar to rice or couscous) it is actually a seed of a leafy plant, related to spinach and Swiss chard. Those preparing it for the first time often complain that it is too mushy. The secret is to bring it to a rolling boil and then take it off the heat. Keep it covered and stir occasionally as it cools down.

You can enjoy it for breakfast, lunch, in side dishes, dinner and even in desserts. Given its "it food" status, quinoa is readily available and should be considered a pantry essential.

The Practice: Breakfast is exactly as it sounds: we 'break the fast' from not eating while we sleep. Yoga is the invitation for us to fast from what no longer services so that we may embrace our true nature by becoming the practice. Like the "break fast" quinoa symbolizes the ending of a period of time and the beginning of a new day, each pose must end so that we may begin one. Before each pose we return to the breath as a way to release that which is in the past and embrace what is the present.

Breathing Meditation Instruction: Sit in a comfortable position. Relax and place the hands lightly on the knees. Close your eyes and begin to breathe. Be mindful of inhales and exhales. Begin to count each breath. And as you breathe create a mantra that incorporates your intention. "I breathe this breath for the preparation of this meal. I am aware of the Universe. This food and breath are one."

Happy Baby Pose (Ananda Balasana) Instruction: A stress reliever and gentle way to stretch the back, Happy Baby is a lovely way to greet the day. Lie flat on your back and draw your knees into your chest. Reach down and grab the outsides of your feet. Make sure to square your feet toward the ceiling. If you cannot reach your feet make sure you hold a strap that is draped across the balls of your feet so that knees are forming a 90-degree angle or are perpendicular to the floor. Remain in this pose for 90 seconds.

Breakfast Quinoa

2 CUPS QUINOA

3 CUPS VEGETABLE STOCK

I CUP ONION, CHOPPED

I CUP RED BELL PEPPER, CHOPPED

I CUP CANDIED GINGER, CHOPPED

2 CUPS DRIED FRUIT, CHOPPED (AN ASSORTMENT OF APRICOTS, CRANBERRIES, CHERRIES AND BLUEBERRIES WORKS NICELY)

I CUP SLICED ALMONDS

MINT FOR GARNISH

Bring quinoa and vegetable broth to a hard rolling boil. Remove from heat and cover, fluffing with a fork every 10 minutes until all of the liquid is absorbed and it has cooled down.

Mix together remaining ingredients and toss with maple syrup balsamic dressing (below). Garnish with mint. Serves 6 to 8.

Maple Balsamic Vinaigrette

2 CLOVES GARLIC, FINELY CHOPPED

2 TABLESPOONS DIJON MUSTARD

I TABLESPOON MAPLE SYRUP

6 TABLESPOONS BALSAMIC VINEGAR

I CUP OLIVE OIL

FRESH GROUND PEPPER

Whisk all ingredients together and let stand for 1 hour.

Quinoa Salad

This salad packs a powerful punch beyond the protein-rich quinoa. Mung bean sprouts are low in calories, contain fiber and B vitamins, and deliver a boost of vitamins C and K. Pine nuts are nutrient-rich, offering health-promoting antioxidant benefits. Chives contain calcium and tomatoes are legendary in supporting heart health.

2 CUPS QUINOA

4 CUPS VEGETABLE STOCK

2 LARGE TOMATOES, CHOPPED

1 LARGE BUNCH CHIVES, CHOPPED

1/2 CUP YOUNG MUNG BEAN SPROUTS

1/2 CUP RAW PINE NUTS

Dressing:

1/3 CUP OLIVE OIL OR WALNUT OIL

1 LIME OR MEYER LEMON, JUICED

2 CLOVES GARLIC, MINCED

PINCH SEA SALT

Bring quinoa and vegetable broth to a boil. Cover; reduce heat to simmer for 10 to 15 minutes. While quinoa is cooking, chop tomatoes and chives. Mix dressing. Remove quinoa from heat. Allow to cool. Fluff quinoa and add vegetables and pine nuts. Gently mix dressing into quinoa mixture. Serve cold or warm. Serves 6.

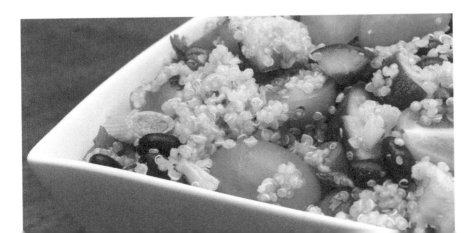

The Practice: The Quinoa Salad is absolute perfection. Quinoa, the center of this creation, is considered a perfect protein. Shamatha Vipashyana Meditation is done with soul or singular purposes to see the truth of what is real. As we dive into this expression, we take the time to know our own perfection.

Shamatha Vipashyana Meditation Instruction: Find a comfortable place where you can be still and uninterrupted. Sit with your legs crossed, upright and with your eyes open. Become aware of your breathing. Notice when the breath moves in and out of the body. Stay with your breathing and heed the expansion of your lungs and chest as you breathe in and the contraction as you exhale. Continue to sit and breathe until you reach that precious moment of clarity of who you are. You will see your perfection. Continue this practice each day for 21 days, until it becomes a ritual.

Quinoa Risotto

Mushrooms contain some of the most potent natural medicines. In order to fully benefit from the mushroom's compelling properties, opt for organic whenever possible. This risotto is rich, flavorful and filling and the mushroom flavor carries through each savory bite.

1 CUP QUINOA
1 TABLESPOON OLIVE OIL
1 CUP ONION, CHOPPED
3 CLOVES GARLIC, MINCED
1 CUP VEGETABLE BROTH
1 CUP ALMOND MILK
8 OUNCES MUSHROOMS, SLICED
3/4 CUP PARMESAN CHEESE OR NUTRITIONAL YEAST

Rinse and drain quinoa 3 times, using a fine mesh strainer to remove the bitter outer coating. Heat olive oil in a heavy saucepan or Dutch oven over medium-high heat. Add onion and cook until soft, stirring constantly. Add garlic and quinoa and continue stirring a minute or two. Stir in broth and milk. Bring to a boil, and then reduce heat to low and simmer until quinoa is tender, stirring occasionally, approximately 10–12 minutes. Add mushrooms and cook another 3-5 minutes, stirring often. Remove from heat. Add cheese or nutritional yeast and let stand a few minutes, so risotto can thicken. Serves 2 to 4.

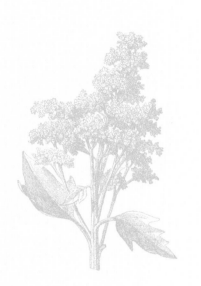

The Practice: Risotto is the quintessential Italian dish. Not unlike yoga, Italy is known for its warriors. In yoga practice you'll encounter Warrior 1, 2 and 3, Reverse Warrior and Exalted Warrior. As we create a dish that honors strength and power, we invite you to connect with the Warrior within you.

Warrior One Pose (Virabhadrasana One) Instruction: The Warrior pose cultivates the qualities of a warrior — honesty, righteousness, standing up for justice. Stand tall and focused on your mat. Step the left leg back into a long leg lunge and turn the foot diagonal to the left corner. Deepen the front knee to a 45-degree bend and reach the arms strong overhead.

Quinoa Tabouli

2 CUPS QUINOA, COOKED
1 CUP PARSLEY, CHOPPED
1/2 CUP SCALLIONS, CHOPPED
2 TABLESPOONS MINT
2 TABLESPOONS BASIL
3 GARLIC CLOVES, MINCED
JUICE OF 1 LEMON
1/4 CUP OLIVE OIL
SALT AND PEPPER TO TASTE
1/4 CUP OLIVES, SLICED

Place all ingredients in a mixing bowl and toss together lightly. Chill for 1 hour or more to allow flavors to blend. Garnish with olives. Serves 4.

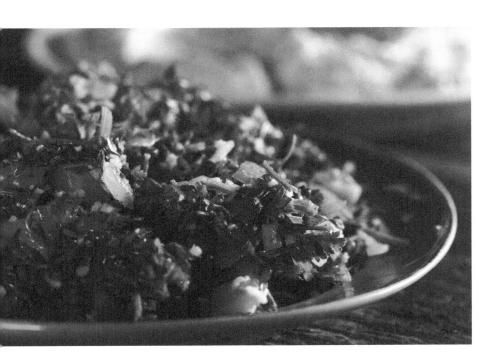

The Practice: Traditionally tabouli (also spelled tabbouleh) is an Arab salad filled with Mediterranean delights. When exploring the connection of tabouli and yoga, we are reminded of what yoga is all about — the practice of seeing the Oneness of two things that appear to be separate. When connecting India and the Middle East, what better way than to do so with food and yoga. It takes practice to experience the Oneness Consciousness. We must begin to see what cultures have in common instead of what separates us.

Thread the Needle Pose (Parsva Balasana) Instruction: If you have stiffness and pain, this pose can provide relief by stretching and opening the shoulders, chest, arms, upper back and neck. It releases the tension that is commonly held in the upper back between the shoulder blades. This pose also provides a mild twist to the spine, which further reduces tension. Begin on all fours (table pose), with hands shoulder-width apart. Turn the right palm upwards and thread the right hand underneath the left arm. Bring the right shoulder and the right side of the face toward the floor. Rest on the right cheek for three long breaths. Bring the left arm up off the floor and send it straight up toward the ceiling, releasing the left shoulder. Bend the left elbow and see if you can reach around to hold your waist or the right thigh. Stay here for six to twelve breaths. To get out of the pose, plant your left hand firmly on the ground and use the weight of it and return to table pose. Repeat on the other side.

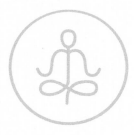

The Practice: Quinoa and seitan are each an independently perfect source of protein. They could happily and effectively stand alone but when combined, they offer an explosion of great taste. It reminds us of the saying, "some things are better done with someone else." Group practice is the same way. We could do Butterfly Pose at home by ourselves, but it is so much more fun with a group of practitioners holding that pose simultaneously in one accord. If you are a home yogi, it might be time for you to step out of your box and experience the collective.

Butterfly Pose (Badhakonasana) Instruction: Sit with your spine erect and legs spread straight out. Bend your knees and bring the soles of your feet together. Interlace your hands around your feet. Begin to gently slap both legs up and down, like the wings of a butterfly. Start slowly and gradually increase the speed. While practicing Butterfly Pose, create a mantra or chant that states you are whole and renewed. "I am whole, renewed and complete now."

Seitan and Quinoa Salad

Seitan is a popular vegetarian meat substitute that's been prepared in Asian countries for generations. It's derived from the protein portion of whole wheat and you'll find it stands in nicely in a variety of meat recipes. And seitan has more protein than either tofu or tempeh and is a staple for many vegetarians.

2 CUPS QUINOA
3 CUPS VEGETABLE STOCK
SALT TO TASTE
1 CUP PINE NUTS, TOASTED
4 TABLESPOONS RED WINE VINEGAR
PEPPER TO TASTE
4 TABLESPOONS OLIVE OIL
3 CUPS COOKED SEITAN, FINELY CHOPPED (RECIPE FOLLOWS)
1 1/2 CUPS GREEN AND RED GRAPES, QUARTERED

Bring quinoa and vegetable stock to a hard rolling boil. Remove from heat and cover, fluffing with a fork every 10 minutes until all of the liquid is absorbed and it has cooled down. Whisk vinegar and oil. Add seitan, grapes, pine nuts and quinoa. Toss well and add salt and pepper to taste. Serves 4.

Grilled Seitan

8-OUNCE PIECE OF SEITAN
POULTRY SEASONING
2 TABLESPOONS OLIVE OIL

Mix olive oil and poultry seasoning. Add seitan and let marinate for 1 hour. Preheat grill to medium heat. Grill for 4 to 5 minutes, until slightly charred. Flip and cook the other side for 4 to 5 minutes.

Black Bean and Lime Quinoa

3 CUPS WATER OR VEGETABLE STOCK
JUICE AND ZEST FROM 3 LIMES
2 TABLESPOONS OLIVE OIL
1 TABLESPOON VEGETABLE OIL
1 CUP QUINOA
1 (15-OUNCE) CAN BLACK BEANS, RINSED AND DRAINED
2 MEDIUM TOMATOES, DICED
4 SCALLIONS, CHOPPED
3 CLOVES GARLIC
1/4 CUP FRESH CILANTRO, CHOPPED
SALT AND PEPPER TO TASTE

Whisk together lime zest and juice, oils, salt, pepper in a large bowl. In a medium-sized pot cover the quinoa with the water or vegetable stock and bring to a boil, about 15 minutes. Cover and remove from heat and let sit until all of the water or stock is absorbed. Cut vegetables while you wait. When liquid is absorbed, fluff with a fork and toss in the bowl with the lime zest dressing and add the black beans, tomatoes, scallions and garlic. Season with salt and pepper to taste and garnish with cilantro.
Serves 4 to 6.

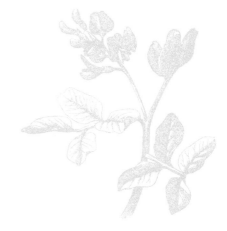

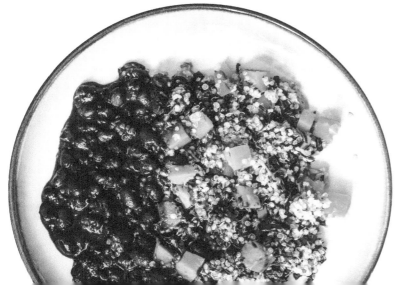

The Practice: Side dish or main course, Black Bean and Lime Quinoa can be enjoyed either way. Yoga is similar in that it can be your complete physical practice or it can be a satisfying side dish to a physical practice you may already have in place. You can decide how to best incorporate yoga into your life by engaging in a contemplative meditation. Go within during meditation and ask the simple question "Is yoga my only practice?" or "What is it that my body needs?" Once you have asked the question have faith that you will receive the answer. Self-exploration is one of the main principles of yoga; know thyself.

Curried Quinoa

Curry powder is famously known for its anti-inflammatory and antioxidant properties. In addition to the health benefits this dish is a textural delight. The crunch of slivered almonds, the chewy raisins, the snap of green peppers and the sweetness of the peas offer a pleasing and harmonious dance on the palate while the quinoa satisfies the need for protein.

2 CUPS QUINOA

4 CUPS WATER

1/2 CUP SLIVERED ALMONDS, TOASTED

1/2 CUP RAISINS

2 LARGE TOMATOES

4 CARROTS, GRATED

1 CUP SWEET PEAS

1 GREEN BELL PEPPER

4 TEASPOONS CURRY POWDER

2 TEASPOONS CHILI POWDER

1 TEASPOON CUMIN

1/2 CUP CILANTRO, CHOPPED

KOSHER SALT

In a good-sized pot sauté quinoa kernels in a little bit of olive oil for 4 minutes, then pour in water, cover and let boil 15 minutes until absorbed. Cut up vegetables while you wait. When water is absorbed, fluff with a fork and add spices, vegetables (except for shredded carrots and cilantro), almonds and raisins. After stirring a good 30 seconds on heat, remove, dish into bowls, and garnish with carrots and cilantro. Serves 4 to 6.

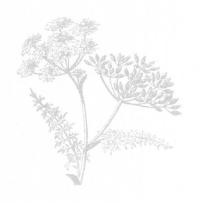

The Practice: Quinoa is a fairly mild and bland grain until it's seasoned. Curry is a hot spicy powder that you would likely not eat on its own. Separately they don't work, but together they are the culinary Yin-Yang, balancing each other perfectly. Yoga is all about recognizing the balance. In a twisting lunge, you can feel the battle between stretching and strengthening. While one side is stretching the other side is releasing into a deep stretch until finally there is a realization that there is no battle at all, just the expression of pure balance.

Twisting Side-angle Pose (Parsvakonasana) Instruction: Coming from Warrior 1, place the hands into Namaste, also known as Anjali mudra (AHN-jah-lee MOO-dra), the praying hands position (hands over the heart). Lift the torso and twist toward the opposite side of the body, crossing the elbow over the knee, continuing to expand the twist by looking toward the sky.

Quinoa Burger

1 1/2 CUPS COOKED QUINOA
1 CUP HUMMUS
2 TABLESPOONS TOMATO PASTE
1 TABLESPOON SESAME OIL
1 TABLESPOON SOY SAUCE
10 BASIL LEAVES, CHOPPED
2 SPRIGS THYME, CHOPPED
PINCH CAYENNE PEPPER TO TASTE
SALT AND PEPPER TO TASTE
6 BURGER BUNS
MIXED GREENS TO DRESS BURGER
AVJAR SAUCE

Blend all ingredients in a bowl or food processor. Divide burger mix into 6 equal portions and form into 4-inch patties. Grill on medium heat 5 minutes each side, until browned and firm. Place patties on buns and top with avjar and mixed greens. Serves 6.

Homemade Avjar

8-12 FRESH RED PAPRIKA (MILD OR MEDIUM-HOT, TO TASTE)
4 MEDIUM-SIZE EGGPLANTS
1/2 CUP OLIVE OIL
1 LARGE ONION, MINCED
3 LARGE GARLIC CLOVES, CHOPPED
JUICE OF 1 LEMON
1/4 CUP PARSLEY LEAVES
SALT AND PEPPER TO TASTE

Roast the paprika and eggplants in a preheated 475°F oven until the skin is blistered and darkened, approximately 30 minutes. Remove from oven and place the now roasted vegetables in a paper bag and let them steam in their own heat for 10 minutes. Peel off and discard the burnt skin along with the stems and seeds. Mash the peppers and eggplant pulp together to form a slightly chunky mass. You can do this with a fork or in a food processor. Heat 3 tablespoons of oil in a large skillet and sauté the onion until very soft. Add garlic and cook for 2 more minutes. Remove from the heat and stir in the pepper-eggplant pulp, mixing well. Slowly drizzle the remaining oil into the mixture, stirring constantly to incorporate all of the oil. Add the lemon juice, parsley, and salt and pepper to taste.

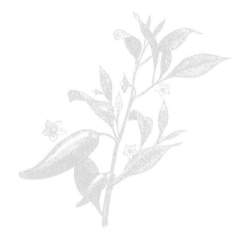

The Practice: This quinoa burger is a real treat. We often associate burgers with a casual gathering of family and friends and the informal joy that accompanies eating something a little messy with our hands. It is so important to enjoy life and indulge in the delights the Universe has in store for us. We must be willing to take the time to experience what we love when it comes to food and when it comes to yoga. What's your favorite pose? What's your favorite type of yoga? Who is your favorite yoga instructor? The practice is simple; approach your practice as if it were an expression of joy. Do what you love. To know what practice activates happiness, you must be willing to get out there and explore. Exploration is a practice. To know thyself you must be willing to take an adventure within.

The Practice: Mix Berry Quinoa Pudding is richly satisfying while remaining a healthy dessert, tasty and low in calories. The practice is to enjoy every bite of the pudding treat that will empower and energize you before and after your yoga practice. Be mindful of the food you eat. Choose the highest nutrients with the most pleasurable punch when feeding the body temple. Remember, you are worth the best and your practice deserves the best fuel possible.

Lotus Flower Mudra: Mudras are gestures or positions, usually of the hands, that influence or guide energy flow, relax the brain and can alter mood. We can talk to the body through mudras for healing and intention-setting. Lotus Flower Mudra is a good finger stretcher. Bring your hands together in the prayer pose near the heart, thumbs lightly touching the chest. Touch together the pinkies, palms of the hand and the thumbs to create a lotus flower blossom. Inhale and bring your hands up to the ceiling. Keep the palms of your hands, pinkies and thumbs touching. Spread your three middle fingers as wide as possible. Now exhale and bring your hands back to prayer pose, pressing the palms together near the chest. Let the elbows come out to the side and press your hands together. Inhale and repeat, bringing your hands into the Lotus mudra. Exhale back into prayer pose. Repeat this process ten times while you imagine welcoming the goodness of the universe into your heart.

Mix Berry Quinoa Pudding

2 CUPS ALMOND MILK

I CUP QUINOA

2 CUPS MIXTURE BLACKBERRIES, BLUEBERRIES, STRAWBERRIES, RASPBERRIES

I/2 TEASPOON GROUND CINNAMON

I/3 CUP CHOPPED PECANS, TOASTED

4 TEASPOONS AGAVE NECTAR

Combine almond milk and quinoa in a medium saucepan. Bring to a boil over high heat. Reduce heat to medium-low; cover and simmer 15 minutes or until most of the liquid is absorbed. Turn off heat; let stand covered 5 minutes. Stir in berries and cinnamon; transfer to 4 bowls and top with pecans. Drizzle 1 teaspoon agave nectar over each serving. Serves 4.

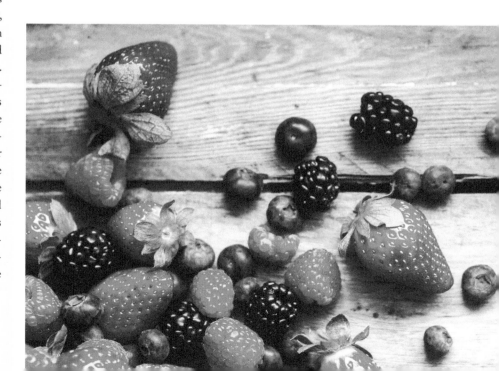

Quinoa Orange and Cranberry Cookies

1 1/2 CUPS WHITE WHOLE WHEAT FLOUR
  (RICE FLOUR OR GLUTEN-FREE ARE OPTIONS)
1 TEASPOON KOSHER SALT
1/2 TEASPOON BAKING POWDER
1/2 TEASPOON BAKING SODA
1 STICK BUTTER, ROOM TEMPERATURE
1/4 CUP SUGAR
1/4 CUP (PACKED) LIGHT BROWN SUGAR
1/4 CUP MAPLE SYRUP
2 LARGE EGGS
1 TEASPOON VANILLA
1/2 TEASPOON ALMOND EXTRACT
1 CUP COOKED QUINOA, COOLED
1 CUP OLD-FASHIONED OATS
1 CUP DRIED CRANBERRIES (ORANGE-FLAVORED IF YOU CAN FIND THEM)
ZEST OF 1 ORANGE
1/2 CUP SLIVERED ALMONDS

Preheat oven to 375°F. Line 2 baking sheets with parchment paper. Whisk flour, salt, baking powder and baking soda in a medium bowl. Using an electric mixer, beat butter, both sugars and syrup in a large bowl until light and fluffy, about 3 minutes. Add eggs, almond extract, vanilla and beat until pale and fluffy, about 2 minutes. Beat in flour mixture, 1/2 cup at a time. Stir in quinoa, oats, cranberries, orange zest and almonds. Spoon dough in 2-tablespoon portions onto prepared sheets, spacing 1 inch apart. Bake cookies until golden, 12–15 minutes. Transfer cookies to a wire rack and let cool. Makes 4 dozen.

The Practice: Yoga is like a cookie — one offering rarely satisfies. A really good cookie can creep into your consciousness. Yoga is the same. When you have connected with the practice and you have experienced the "yoga joy" it will not leave you alone. It calls your spirit. The body, mind and soul not only require the practice, but they start to crave yoga when there is a yoga void. Listen to the yoga craving. When it calls your name, act upon it. Get into action. Get moving. The desire to practice and move is no mistake or coincidence. It is an invitation.

Cat Cow Stretch (Chakravakasana): Cat pose is often paired with Cow pose for a gentle warm-up sequence. When practiced together the poses help to stretch the body and prepare it for other activity. It's a great flow that heats up the spine and abs, and strengthens the back when practiced consistently. Begin on all fours — table pose — with hand right below and shoulders and knees right below the hips with a neutral spine. On the inhale, drop your belly while your abdominal muscles hug the spine. Take your gaze upward toward the ceiling. Let the movement in the spine start from your tailbone so that your neck is the last body part to move. On the next exhale round your spine toward the ceiling. Drop your head and take your gaze to your navel. Repeat the cat-cow stretch on each inhale and exhale, matching the movement to your breath. Continue for five to ten breaths, moving the whole spine during the sequence. After your final exhale return to neutral spine.

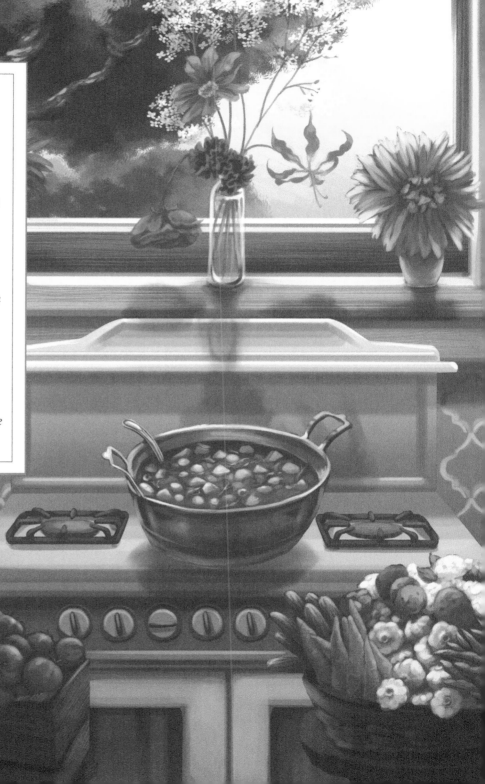

Soups

Soup is the quintessential healing food. It's also the ideal "go-to" when you're not feeling like a big meal, yet want something flavor- and nutri-ent-packed. A pot of soup simmering on the stove evokes a sense of home, a sense of well-being. The ultimate in comfort and nurturing, soup can also stimulate creative expression. Very few dishes offer the flexibility and ease of soup. And soups can be en-joyed warm or cool, depending on the needs and desires of the body temple.

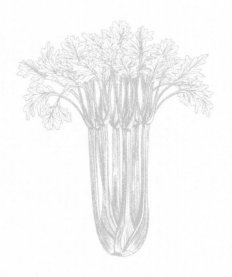

The Practice: When a recipe requires a lot of chopping we have to stand tall with a strong core. Mountain pose delivers the core strength to face many of life's challenges. Harness the qualities of the pose while prepping your soup stock. Strength. Power. Longevity. Height. These are the qualities of your divine self. As you stand tall and prepare this dish, connect with the mountain strength that is your life.

Mountain Pose (Tadasana) Instruction: Stand tall at the top of your mat, feet hip-distance apart, spread the toes to create a strong base. Draw the shoulders away from the ears and open the arms while spreading your fingers.

Everything But the Kitchen Sink Vegetable Stock

The beauty of a good vegetable stock is that you can use any combination of vegetables and herbs that you may prefer — or have on hand. It can lack the "richness" of a traditional stock, so we lovingly lace it with seasoning. One way to bring in some of the missing layers and deepen the aromatic notes is to roast the vegetables before simmering them. To do so, toss the vegetables liberally in olive oil and generously dress with salt and pepper. Roast in a 425°F oven for about 1 1/2 hours. You can even roast in batches so you don't crowd the baking pan. Follow the basic recipe below, or if you are like us at *The Lotus Kitchen* you can collect all of your vegetable scraps (including the onion skins for a nice rich color) for variance and convenience. We simply gather them in a stockpot and refrigerate until we have enough (about 6–8 cups) and are ready to use them.

Feel free to add any herbs you have laying around in the last 15 minutes of simmering. You can add ginger, lemongrass and dried Chinese mushrooms and even a kiss of miso for an Asian flair. For a Mexican feel, add diced jalapeño or Serrano chilies and lots of fresh cilantro. The magic of this recipe is you really can't go wrong and it is so much fun to play with your food.

4 CARROTS, CHOPPED

4 CELERY STALKS, CHOPPED (INCLUDING LEAVES)

3 TOMATOES, CHOPPED

1 MEDIUM SWEET POTATO, PEELED AND CHOPPED

1 SCALLION, CHOPPED

1 RED ONION, CHOPPED

6 CLOVES GARLIC, CHOPPED

JUICE OF 1 LEMON

1/2 TEASPOON SALT

1/2 TEASPOON PEPPER

1 TEASPOON THYME

1 BAY LEAF

1 TEASPOON HERBS DE PROVENCE

1/4 TEASPOON CAYENNE PEPPER

1/2 CUP WHITE WINE OR RED WINE FOR A DEEPER COLOR (OR ELIMINATE IF YOU PREFER NOT COOKING WITH WINE)

12 CUPS WATER

In a large soup pot combine all ingredients and bring to a boil over medium heat. Reduce heat and cover and simmer for 1 hour. Strain the stock and toss the solids. You will have approximately 10 cups of stock. You can freeze half for use at a later time. Or you can freeze in ice cube trays and pop out single servings as needed for sauces.

The Lotus Kitchen

Raw Thai Coconut Soup

Thai cooking is lively and aromatic and this soup is no exception. The coconut, ginger and garlic play nicely off the heat of the peppers. It's at once complex and simple, not unlike a vibrant yoga practice.

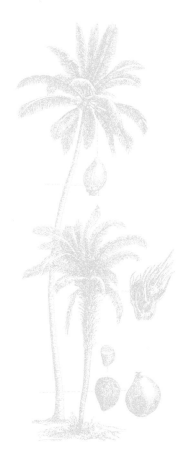

2 YOUNG COCONUTS

1 CUP CHERRY TOMATOES

1 AVOCADO

1 CLOVE GARLIC, PEELED

1/2 INCH FRESH GINGER, PEELED

1 TEASPOON MUSTARD POWDER

1/2 TEASPOON SEA SALT

2 TABLESPOONS SOY SAUCE

JUICE OF 2 LIMES

3 RED THAI CHILI PEPPERS

Garnish:

1 CUP CILANTRO, CHOPPED

2 CUPS TOMATOES, DICED

1/3 CUP RED ONION, DICED

Slice the coconuts in half and pour the juice into a large bowl. Scoop out the flesh and place in the bowl. Liquefy all ingredients with an immersion blender. Pour into bowl and garnish with cilantro, tomato and onion before serving. You can also use a traditional blender by placing all of the ingredients and liquefying. Serve room temperature. Serves 4.

The Practice: Soup that is cool to the touch but heats presents opposition; once you taste it you will know true balance.

Yoga Balance: Some think our mind and body are separate, but as we practice yoga we learn to yoke our body and mind together. That is the main intention of the yoga practice. Recognize that you are one with your mind and body in all of your practice.

Raw Fresh Okra Gazpacho

Okra brings a lovely sheen to dishes where it's front and center, and it is known for its role in healthy digestion. High in fiber and vitamin C, it is also a fine source of calcium and potassium. The Thai chilies bring a nice heat to the chilled gazpacho, a lovely juxtaposition that awakens the senses.

2 CUPS FRESH OKRA
2 CUPS FRESH TOMATOES
1 CUP ONION
1 CUP CUCUMBER
1 LARGE GARLIC CLOVE
1/3 OLIVE OIL
JUICE OF 2 LEMONS
1/2 TEASPOON THAI CHILIES, MINCED
1/2 CUP CILANTRO, CHOPPED
1/3 CUP PARSLEY, CHOPPED
4 CUPS TOMATO JUICE

Place first 5 ingredients into the bowl of a food processor fitted with the steel blade. Turn to chop and dice setting and begin to puree. While processing, pour in the olive oil and lemon juice. Then add the cilantro and parsley. Lastly add tomato juice and puree briefly to a chunky consistency. Refrigerate and serve chilled. Serves 4.

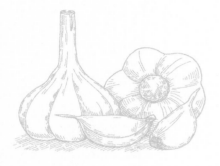

The Practice: Like the tomato, said to heal all of our sufferings and maladies, yoga is a healing practice. We must think of our practice as healing for the mind, body, and spirit. As you eat the tomatoes in the gazpacho, feel the vibration of healing. Upward-Facing Dog Pose is the posture that opens the heart chakra, allowing the heart to heal. The ability to love and receive love is magnified.

Upward-Facing Dog Pose (Urdvha Mukha Svanasana) Instruction: Lay flat on the mat, stomach down in prone position. Place hands flat on the floor under the arms. Press the hands into the floor and straighten the arms. Drop the shoulders from the ears, and lift the hips off the floor, keeping the legs straight, keeping the feet flat connected to the mat.

Party Miso Soup

For over 2,500 years miso has been a staple in Chinese and Japanese diets, where many greet the day with a warm bowl of miso to energize their bodies and stimulate digestion. Miso is a powerful detoxifier containing essential amino acids, making it a complete protein. You can prepare this soup for a crowd or you can store it in the refrigerator and enjoy a hot cup in the morning before you commence your yoga practice.

8 CUPS WATER
1 INCH FRESH GINGER, FINELY CHOPPED
1 CUP SHIRO MISO (A FERMENTED SOYBEAN PASTE)
BUNCH OF SCALLIONS, THINLY SLICED
1 CUP FIRM TOFU, CHOPPED INTO 1/4-INCH CUBES

Bring 7 1/2 cups of water and ginger to a boil. Whisk miso and 1/2 cup water in a small bowl until smooth and whisk into soup. Add tofu and scallions and simmer for a few minutes before serving. Serves 8 to 10.

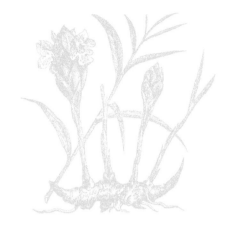

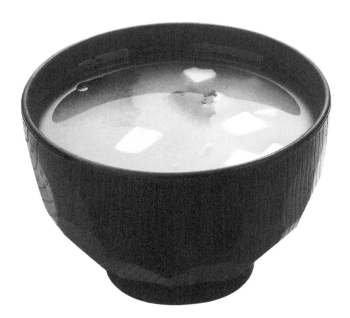

The Practice: The healing properties of miso bring you back to a state of equilibrium as does the classic yoga pose Downward-Facing Dog. It is a perfect pose to rest, so we may begin again. When the practice brings you to fatigue, remember Downward-Facing Dog and the perfect equilibrium.

Downward-Facing Dog Pose (Adho Mukha Svanasana) Instruction: From a kneeling position place hands and feet on the mat and lift the hips toward the sky to create the perfect upside down V shape. Hands should be shoulder-width apart and feet hip-width apart, spreading fingers and toes to create a strong base. While practicing Downward-Facing Dog, create a mantra or chant that states that you are whole and renewed. Create an affirmation that affirms your healing is taking place now. For example: "My body knows how to heal itself and I am open and will allow it to be."

Crowd-Pleasing Minestrone

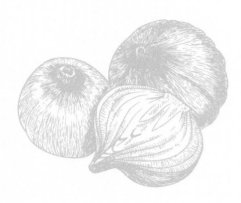

2 TABLESPOONS OLIVE OIL

2 YELLOW ONIONS, DICED

6 STALKS CELERY (INCLUDING LEAVES), THINLY SLICED

3 CARROTS, CHOPPED

1 TABLESPOON ITALIAN HERBS (DRIED BLEND OF OREGANO, PARSLEY, BASIL, ROSEMARY, THYME)

Sauté above ingredients over medium heat in large soup pot, then cover to sweat for five minutes.

Uncover and add:

4 CLOVES GARLIC, MINCED

Sauté 5 more minutes, then add:

12 CUPS VEGETABLE STOCK

1 BOX CHOPPED TOMATOES OR 3 CUPS CANNED CHOPPED TOMATOES

2 YUKON GOLD POTATOES, DICED

2 (15-OUNCE) CANS CANNELLINI BEANS, DRAINED

1 SMALL HEAD SAVOY CABBAGE, QUARTERED AND SLICED

Bring to boil and simmer 30 minutes. Then add:

8 OUNCES PASTA OF YOUR CHOICE

6 MORE CUPS VEGETABLE BROTH

2 CUPS GREEN BEANS, CUT INTO 1-INCH PIECES

Simmer 15 minutes. Serve with freshly grated Parmesan cheese. Serves 12.

The Practice: The Karma Yoga practice is the act of serving others. This crowd-pleasing soup serves many. When serving this dish focus on how you may serve the universe and others to better the planet. Like a breathing meditation that helps one to connect with the universe, Karma Yoga serves as a reminder that we are all connected.

Breathing Meditation Instruction: Sit in a comfortable position. Relax and place the hands lightly on the knees. Close your eyes and begin to breathe. Be mindful of your inhale and your exhale. Begin to count each breath. As you breathe create a mantra that incorporates your intention. "I breathe this breath for the preparation of this meal. I am aware of the Universe. This food and breath are one."

Sweet Beet Soup

Beets are a gorgeous gift for the body temple. Ruby red, this jewel from the earth provides an energy boost, purifies the blood, offers tryptophan to nurture mental health and contains vitamins A and C and niacin. Beets are available year-round and this soup is a colorful way to nourish guests and self.

1 TABLESPOON OLIVE OIL
2 MEDIUM RED ONIONS
1 (4-INCH) PIECE FRESH GINGER, PEELED
6 CLOVES GARLIC, PEELED
8 CUPS VEGETABLE STOCK
2 POUNDS BEETS
2 POUNDS CARROTS
PINCH OF KOSHER SALT
1/2 TEASPOON WHITE PEPPER

Roughly chop the carrots, beets, red onions, peeled ginger and garlic. Toss with olive oil and place on sheet pan. Sprinkle with salt and pepper and roast for about 1 hour until tender. Move to soup pot and add the stock. Simmer over medium heat until the carrots are tender. Puree and season with salt and pepper. Serves 6.

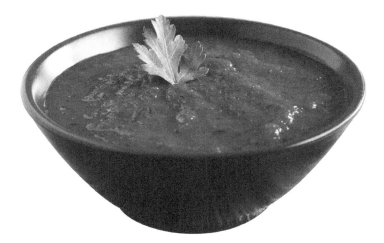

The Practice: Beets are also a top source of nitrates, which when converted to nitric oxide actually expands veins and arteries, allowing more blood to flow and carry oxygen to the brain. This makes beets a perfect wisdom food. Yoga stimulates the mind and creates clarity in one's life. The Hatha Yoga pose shoulder stand or any inverted pose is for brain health. The upside down pose allows oxygen to flow to the brain, while releasing pressure from the legs. Shoulder stand is an excellent yoga pose. Like the beets it nourishes the brain with well-needed oxygen and rich blood flow.

Shoulder Stand Pose (Salamba Sarvangasana) Instruction: Lie flat on your mat and breathe easy. Place both feet flat on the floor, hip-width apart with toes facing forward. Tuck your chin toward the chest and place your hands to the side of the body on the floor. Lift your hips and knees to the sky; raise your hands to your lumbar spine. Steady your body by placing the weight of your body onto the elbows and shoulders. When ready, extend the leg toward the sky. While practicing the shoulder stand, visualize the oxygen flowing to the brain with ease and grace. Create a mantra that incorporates the affirmations that the brain is full of oxygen, therefore thoughts are clear.

Roasted Carrot, Asparagus and Ginger Soup

Any time you can hit a dish with fresh ginger is a happy day in The Lotus Kitchen. The sweetness of the carrots in this soup cries for the flavorful balance that ginger delivers — and have you noticed how ginger always seems to make a hot soup seem even warmer? And the fresh asparagus not only delivers a green element, it also adds a richness to the traditional carrot ginger blend.

1 TABLESPOON OLIVE OIL
2 MEDIUM RED ONIONS, SLICED
1 (4-INCH) PIECE FRESH GINGER, PEELED
6 CLOVES GARLIC, PEELED
8 CUPS VEGETABLE STOCK
2 POUNDS CARROTS
2 POUNDS ASPARAGUS
PINCH OF KOSHER SALT
1/2 TEASPOON WHITE PEPPER

Preheat oven to 375°F. Roughly chop the carrots, asparagus, red onions, peeled ginger and garlic. Toss with olive oil and place on sheet pan. Sprinkle with salt and pepper and roast for about one hour until tender. Move to soup pot and add the stock. Simmer over medium heat until the carrots are tender. Puree and season with salt and pepper. Serves 4 to 6.

The Practice: As children we're told to eat our carrots to improve vision. Jnana Yoga is the practice of seeing clearly what is right and what is real. As we dive into this soup, ask the Universe to show you what is real, and what is the illusion you have made up for yourself to protect you from transformation. One pose that allows us to see the truth of our strength is the Warrior Pose. When we stand erect and channel the warrior within, we begin to clearly see our strength. The practice is to see who and what you are. You are a divine being who is strong and full of power.

Warrior One Pose (Virabhadrasana One) Instruction: The Warrior pose cultivates the qualities of a warrior — honesty, righteousness, standing up for justice. Stand tall and focused on your mat. Step the left leg back into a long leg lunge and turn the foot diagonal to the left corner. Deepen the front knee to a 45-degree bend and reach the arms strong over head.

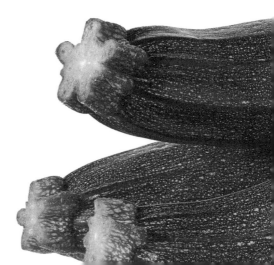

Curry Zucchini Soup

There are many different curries, all rich in distinctive flavors from all parts of the world. The familiar golden yellow powder found in Western culture includes coriander, turmeric, cumin, fenugreek, cinnamon and chili peppers. Ingredients in most curries help ease digestion, burn fat and are rich in anti-oxidants. And the flavor? Like no other.

2 POUNDS ZUCCHINI, DICED
6 GREEN ONIONS, SLICED
4 CUPS VEGETABLE STOCK
2 TABLESPOONS BUTTER OR OLIVE OIL
1 TEASPOON GARAM MASALA
1/2 TEASPOON TURMERIC
1/4 TEASPOON CAYENNE PEPPER
SALT AND PEPPER TO TASTE

In a large stockpot, sauté the zucchini and green onions for 5 minutes over medium heat. Add the remaining ingredients. Simmer for 30 minutes. Puree in batches and return to the pan and heat through. Serves 4 to 6.

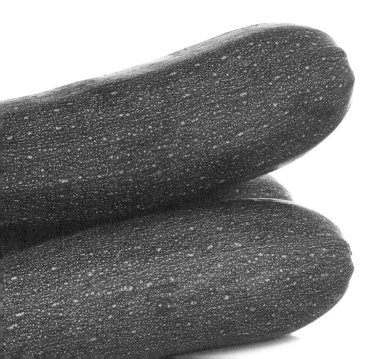

The Practice: The common curry has medicinal uses. It has been used for thousands of years to heat up and cure a variety of ailments from stomach cramps to throat infections. Just as curry heats and heals the body, a principle of yoga called Tapas heats the body through physical practice to purify, cleanse and heal. Set the intention that healing can and will be activated as you taste the delicious meal and participate in the blessed practice. One of the poses that activates healing within is the Wide-legged Forward Bend Pose. It helps to drain the impurities from the body, releasing all the unwanted toxins into the bloodstream so that we may ultimately release them completely from the body. This pose also realigns, rebalances, and soothes your mind and body by calming your energy.

Wide-legged Forward Bend Pose (Padottanasana) Instruction: Spread your legs to a wide straddle position. Slightly bend your knees and hang forward from the hips. Draw in and squeeze your abdominal wall, keeping your hips as high as possible. Place your hands on the floor to support your upper body, releasing your head toward the floor.

Salad

When it comes to salads, The Lotus Kitchen is always open. We enjoy salad for breakfast, lunch, dinner and even as a late-night snack. We love mixing up the greens using a variety of kale, lettuces, chards, spinach and greens. This is another great culinary area to really express creativity and play with all kinds of fruit, vegetable, grain, nut, and legume combinations. And salads allow creativity in plating. Whether you are preparing a salad for one or twenty, take those few extra moments to contemplate presentation. A white plate makes colors pop. Creating a photo-worthy presentation allows the dish to be appreciated by all of the senses. You'll enjoy the salad even more. Mindful eating is more than an awareness of food source, nutrients and flavor harmonizing. It's an aesthetic appreciation as well.

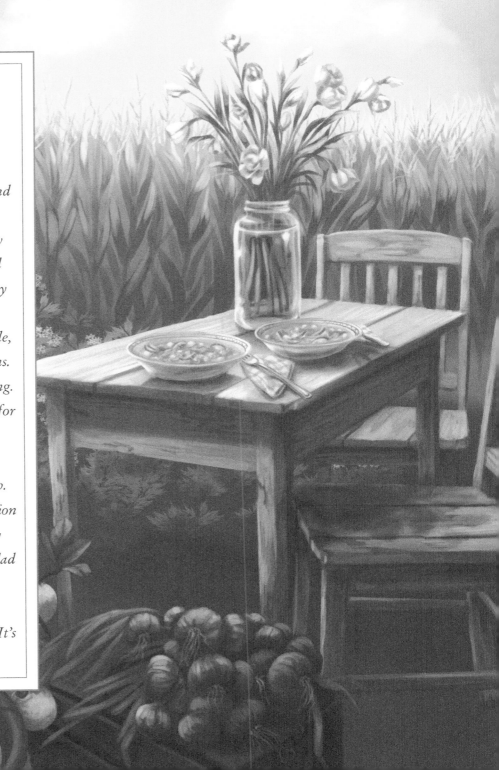

Blueberry Mango Salad

4 LIMES

1 CUP WATER

1/4 CUP AGAVE NECTAR

2 LARGE MANGOS, PEELED AND CUT INTO 1-INCH PIECES

3 CUPS BLUEBERRIES

1/4 CUP CRYSTALLIZED GINGER, FINELY CHOPPED

Remove zest from one lime in strips with a vegetable peeler and cut any white pith from strips with a sharp knife. Squeeze juice from limes. Bring zest, water, and agave to a boil in a saucepan. Remove from heat and stir in lime juice. Let syrup stand 20 minutes, then remove zest with a slotted spoon and discard. Toss together mangoes, blueberries and syrup in a large bowl and sprinkle with ginger. Serves 4.

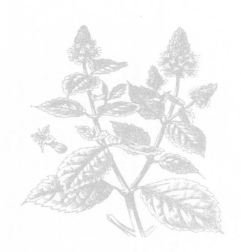

The Practice: The nectar and sweetness of the fruit in this salad remind us that the practice of yoga is sweet nectar as well. When we finish our daily practice of yoga we are reminded of how sweet life is. Physical practice brings us to a place of surrender and final relaxation called Shavasana, the corpse pose. "Life is Good." To get to the nectar of yoga, we must work through the practice. The journey, in this experience, is to recognize the preparation of the salad is very much like the practice of yoga. Once the salad is complete, sit and be still; enjoy every bite. "Life is Good."

Corpse Pose (Savasana) Instruction: We lay on our backs in full rest experiencing the pleasures of the breath and moment. It is also the final meditation of the practice where we remember that life is really really good.

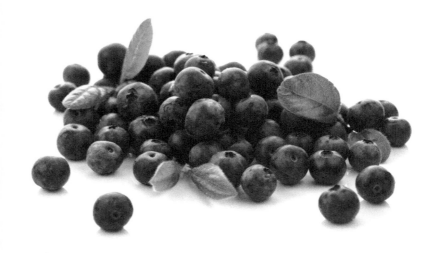

The Lotus Kitchen

Kale Peace Salad

Kale is a powerful addition to soups and stews and is even more enjoyable when baked or sautéed. Many believe it's a little too tough for salad and stay clear of this nutrient-rich leaf. The trick to adding raw kale is to give it a good massage before adding to your salad. Yes, kale needs some love too. A few minutes rubdown will transform a tough, bitter green into a silky and tasty treat. Use a little olive oil, lemon and salt — or a handful of dressing. (Yes, you may use a glove if you prefer.) Remove the fibrous ribs and carefully massage for three to five minutes. Because raw kale is very rich in nutrients it will give you back the love you give it.

1 CUP KALE, FINELY CHOPPED

1 CUP COLLARD GREENS, FINELY CHOPPED

1/2 CUP NAPA CABBAGE, FINELY CHOPPED

1/2 CUP RED CABBAGE, FINELY CHOPPED

1/4 CUP RED ONION, FINELY CHOPPED

1 CUP COOKED BLACK-EYED PEAS, CHILLED

1/2 CUP RAW ALMONDS, FINELY CHOPPED

2 CUPS DRIED CRANBERRIES

Toss together with Orange Vinaigrette:

Clementine Orange Vinaigrette

1/4 CUP CLEMENTINE ORANGE JUICE

ZEST FROM 2 CLEMENTINES

1/2 CUP OLIVE OIL

1/2 CUP BALSAMIC VINEGAR

1/2 CUP MINT LEAVES, DE-STEMMED

Mix ingredients in a blender. Toss with salad, lightly coating. Serves 4 to 6.

The Practice: The peaceful warrior, also known as Warrior 2, is the pose that allows us to make peace with ourselves. While making the Kale Peace Salad, contemplate what in your life needs to be at peace. The characteristic of a peaceful warrior is one who knows what the mission is, and has surrendered to the work of the battle. He or she has made peace within, knowing what needs to be done. What is the work that is called forth from within you?

Warrior Two/Peaceful Warrior (Virabhadrasana Two) Instructions: Warrior 2 or Peaceful Warrior Pose comes from a Warrior 1 position. Turn your back leg to open the foot to match the edges of the outside of the foot with the edges of the back of the mat. Open the torso to face the side of the room, open up arms to shoulder height and anchor both feet to the mat.

Harmonious Lentil Salad

Golden raspberries have a short season — you can find them midsummer with a command performance of a few short weeks in the fall. A little sweeter than traditional red raspberries, they pair nicely with the blood oranges and bring a hint of elegance to brown rice and lentils.

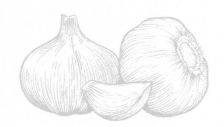

1 CUP LENTILS, COOKED AND CHILLED
1 CUP BROWN RICE, COOKED AND CHILLED
1 PINT GOLDEN RASPBERRIES
2 BLOOD ORANGES, PEELED AND ROUGHLY CHOPPED
1/4 CUP PARSLEY
1/2 CUP GREEN ONIONS

In a large salad bowl toss together and chill for at least 1 hour before serving. Dress with Blood Orange Garlic Vinaigrette. Serves 4.

The Practice: Because our life is so much about going forward and sitting hunched over, the yoga practice is used to bring the body into harmony with itself. The backbend creates balance and harmony within the body, by opening the front, which is naturally forward. The camel pose activates harmony within the body by expanding the anterior part of the body. It is a pose that helps fully stretch the front of the body.

Camel Pose (Ustrasana) Instruction: Begin in a kneeling position with knees at hip-distance apart. Place the back of your hands on the top of the buttocks. Drop your head back without straining the neck, and lift your chest to the sky. Option is to place your hand on the heels of the feet to expand the chest.

Blood Orange Garlic Vinaigrette

Great with the lentil salad, and equally harmonious with a big salad of mixed greens and any vegetables that you have on hand.

2 TABLESPOONS WHITE WINE VINEGAR
1/4 CUP BLOOD ORANGE JUICE
ZEST FROM ONE BLOOD ORANGE
2/3 CUP OLIVE OIL
1 CLOVE GARLIC, FINELY CHOPPED
1 TABLESPOON SHALLOTS, FINELY CHOPPED
2 TEASPOONS FRESH PARSLEY, FINELY CHOPPED
2 TEASPOONS FRESH CHIVES, FINELY CHOPPED
SALT AND PEPPER TO TASTE

Whisk together vigorously. Keeps in the refrigerator for 1 month.

Cucumber Mint Salad

Cucumber water is a staple at many spas and fitness centers. It's a refreshing way to replenish after rigorous play or mindful bodywork. This salad offers refreshment and sustenance, and the mint, cilantro and lime juice combination will soon be one of your favorite blends of flavors.

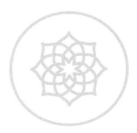

4 CUPS CHOPPED CUCUMBER (3 MEDIUM-SIZED CUCUMBERS)
2 CUPS FRESH MINT LEAVES, DE-STEMMED
1 CUP FRESH CILANTRO, DE-STEMMED
1 CUP LIME JUICE
1/3 CUP GRAPESEED OIL
1 CUP FRESH YELLOW CHERRY TOMATOES
RAW MACADAMIA NUTS, CHOPPED
FRESH BASIL

Combine all ingredients in a large bowl and serve. Serves 4.

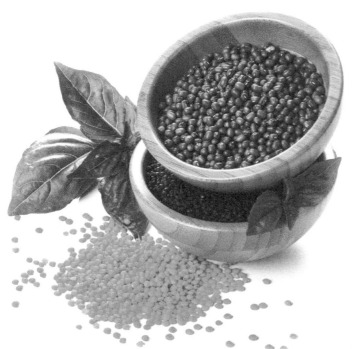

The Practice: The cucumber is the most perfect food for hydration, nutrients and releasing weight. The practice of yoga also helps release weight and unwanted heavy energy. One of the effects of yoga is building heat within, and allowing the body to sweat out everything we do not need. To balance the body, take the time to hydrate with water and cucumbers.

Mindful Eating Practice: This practice is to be aware that the salad is hydrating, nurturing, and creating a healthy body. With each bite be aware of the water of the cucumber that is hydrating the body. Be mindful of each quenching morsel that is blessing your mouth. Feel the energy that the salad is stimulating within the body. The vibration that is delivered from the food is helping to elevate the vibration of the soul. During the ritual create an affirmation that helps remind you that eating is a practice. For example, "I know my mind, body, and spirit are strong as I eat my cucumber salad."

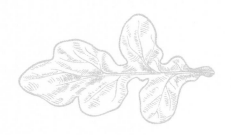

Black Bean and Corn Salad

The heat of the pepper and the briny flavor of the balsamic vinegar make this twist on traditional black bean and corn salad a standout. It's important to use a firmer avocado in this recipe so guacamole won't unintentionally make its way into this zesty dish.

3 CUPS BLACK BEANS (DRAINED AND COOKED AL DENTE)
3 CUPS ROASTED WHITE CORN (COOKED AL DENTE)
1 RED ONION (RAW)
1 RED PEPPER (RAW)
1 CUP CILANTRO
1 GARLIC CLOVE, MINCED
1 JALAPEÑO, MINCED
2 AVOCADOS, CHOPPED (FIRM, NOT OVERLY RIPE)
1/2 CUP OLIVE OIL
1/2 CUP BALSAMIC VINEGAR
1/3 CUP LIME JUICE
ARUGULA LETTUCE

Combine black beans, corn, red pepper, cilantro, jalapeño, and avocado. Add olive oil, vinegar, and lime juice and mix together.

Place on a bed of arugula and serve. Serves 4 to 6.

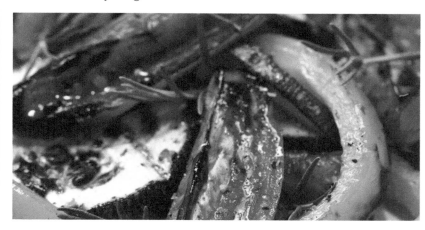

The Practice: Beans and corn sprout goodness. Like a long planting season, after practicing Yoga for a while we begin to see the harvest from our hard work. The sprouts from a practice can be good eating habits, better perception of one's self, and a better awareness of the body. These are all fruits of the labor. Part of crop harvest is the practice of gratitude. Gratitude is the highest appreciation for what is good in your life. After a strong and powerful session of yoga, endorphins are released, which can cause a feeling of euphoria or a sense of gratitude. The practice is to maintain gratitude while preparing this salad. Recognize the harvest of the fruits in your life, and when you sit and partake, be grateful for your life.

The Easy Pose Meditation Instruction: Sitting with your buttocks on the mat, cross your legs with your ankles under your thighs. Rest your hands on your knees, pressing both hips toward the floor. Close your eyes and breathe. Allow your thoughts to open to knowledge and learning. Set the intention to know and feel gratitude.

Grilled Vegetable Platter

A well tended grill is a vegetable's best friend. The key is to lightly char. The difference between a lightly and perfectly charred vegetable and a burnt one can be seconds, not minutes. There are many times we can step away from the oven, grill or stovetop when we are preparing meals. This isn't one of those times. It's mindful cooking and the payoff is a platter of perfectly grilled vegetables that are enhanced with fresh herbs and goat cheese.

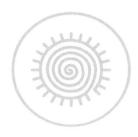

3 RED BELL PEPPERS, SEEDED AND HALVED

3 YELLOW SQUASH, SLICED LENGTHWISE INTO 1/2-INCH-THICK RECTANGLES

3 ZUCCHINI, SLICED LENGTHWISE INTO 1/2-INCH-THICK RECTANGLES

3 JAPANESE EGGPLANT, SLICED LENGTHWISE INTO 1/2-INCH-THICK RECTANGLES

1 BUNCH (1 POUND) ASPARAGUS, TRIMMED

12 GREEN ONIONS

OLIVE OIL

SALT AND PEPPER TO TASTE

3 TABLESPOONS BALSAMIC VINEGAR

2 GARLIC CLOVES, MINCED

1 TEASPOON FRESH ITALIAN PARSLEY LEAVES, CHOPPED

1 TEASPOON FRESH BASIL LEAVES, CHOPPED

1 CUP GOAT CHEESE, CRUMBLED

Place a grill pan over medium-high heat or prepare the barbecue (medium-high heat). Brush the vegetables with oil to coat lightly. Sprinkle the vegetables with salt and pepper. Working in batches, grill the vegetables until tender and lightly charred all over, about 8 to 10 minutes for the bell peppers; 7 minutes for the yellow squash, zucchini, eggplant, 4 minutes for the asparagus and green onions. Arrange the vegetables on a platter. Meanwhile whisk 2 tablespoons of oil, balsamic vinegar, garlic, parsley and basil in a small bowl to blend. Add salt and pepper to taste. Drizzle the herb mixture over the vegetables. Sprinkle with goat cheese and serve. Serves 12.

The Practice: Like the Grilled Veggie Platter, yoga is about the preparation. With the perfect combination of ingredients and preparation, the vegetable platter is a treat that stimulates the love for food. Yoga preparation is a mindset. This is the reason for an opening meditation; it prepares us for a great, delicious practice. Take time to recognize the importance of preparing the body, with the mind. Set our intention for the practice that you choose to have. Sometimes the simple preparation for yoga is breathing. Practice a breath meditation before the preparation of this dish. Just be aware of the breath and set the intention that this will be the best meal ever, and it will be.

Breathing Meditation Instruction: Sit in a comfortable position, relax and lay the hands lightly on the knees. Close the eyes and begin to breathe. Be mindful of when you inhale and when you exhale. Begin to count each breath, and as you breathe create a mantra that incorporates your intention. "I breathe this breath for the preparation of this meal. I am aware of the Universe, this food and the breath are one."

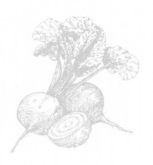

Roasted Beet Salad

1 POUND BEETS, WASHED, STEMS TRIMMED 1/2 INCH ABOVE BEETROOT
1 TABLESPOON HORSERADISH
6 SAGE LEAVES, SLICED
PINCH SALT AND PEPPER
8 OUNCES GOAT CHEESE

Place beets in a tightly covered casserole dish. Pour enough water to cover 1/2 inch at the bottom. Roast at 350°F for 2 1/2 hours. The beets are cooked when the skin is slightly wrinkled and removes easily with your fingers. Remove from oven and as soon as they are cool enough to touch, remove skin and cut into about 8 1/4-inch pieces. While still warm, mix well with horseradish, sage, salt and pepper. Chill for at least 2 hours. Mix well again. Add the crumbled goat cheese. Mix and serve. Serves 6.

The Practice: The beet is a root vegetable that comes from the ground. Yoga is all about grounding. As we prepare and eat the beet salad, this is a time to contemplate what is the force that keeps you grounded, and rooted in all things good. The only thing that grounds us is our connection to something greater. Is it your family, your practice of meditation, or gratitude? Whatever it is, take the time to recognize the force that you are anchored in. Yoga is the practice that anchors and grounds us in a deeper consciousness. Like the beet salad, allow Twisting Side-Angle Pose to ground your awareness that you are one with something bigger than yourself.

Twisting Side-angle Pose (Parsvakonasana) Instruction: Coming from Warrior 1, place the hands into Namaste, also called Anjali mudra (AHN-jah-lee MOO-dra) the hand position (praying hands over the heart). Lift the torso and twist toward the opposite side of the body, crossing the elbow over the knee, continuing to expand the twist by looking toward the sky.

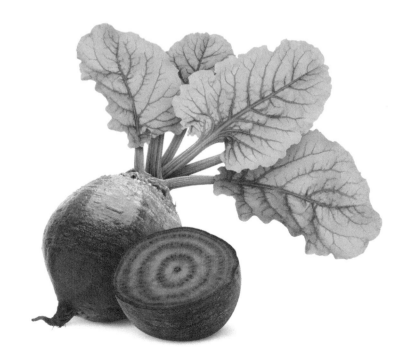

Orzo Salad with Heirloom Tomatoes and Feta

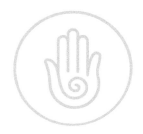

8 OUNCES ORZO

2 TABLESPOONS WHITE WINE VINEGAR

1/2 CUP FRESH LEMON JUICE

1 TEASPOON LEMON ZEST

1/2 CUP OLIVE OIL

1 1/4 POUNDS ASSORTED HEIRLOOM TOMATOES, CUT INTO 1/2-INCH PIECES

1 BUNCH GREEN ONIONS, SLICED

1/2 CUP PITTED OIL-CURED OLIVES, SLICED

1/4 CUP FRESH BASIL, THINLY SLICED

2 TABLESPOONS FRESH ITALIAN PARSLEY, CHOPPED

1 CUP FETA CHEESE, CRUMBLED

Sauté half of the orzo in a little olive oil until golden brown. Cook all of the orzo in large pot of boiling salted water until tender but still firm to bite, stirring occasionally. Drain. Rinse under cold water; drain well. Transfer to medium bowl; cool.

Whisk vinegar and lemon juice in small bowl; gradually whisk in oil. Pour dressing over orzo. Mix in remaining ingredients. Season to taste with salt and pepper. Serves 10.

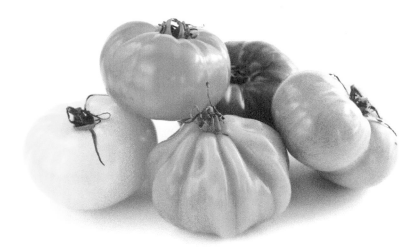

The Practice: Orzo is a pasta, and pasta is unleavened wheat, hard and sometimes dry. The leavening process is a chemical agent used to soften the dough and soften the finished product. What allows us to eat the pasta is a natural leavening that is done by a boiling and heating ceremony. Yoga too is a leavening process — of one's physical self. The practice of heating the body temple is a ceremony that softens one's spirit to allow a mental and emotional transformation to happen. As you prepare the pasta for this amazing dish, feel the softening of your spirit, priming and preparing you for a deeper transformation. One of the poses in yoga that creates a softening process is the Leg Raise. It allows us to be aware of our balance, creating a humbling effect, ultimately softening the ego.

Leg Raise Pose (Padangusthasana) Instruction: Stand tall on the mat and place your hands on your hips. Lift your right knee to hip level and place the hands under the knees. Place the left hand on the left hip and grab the right big toes with the first two fingers and the thumb. A second option is to extend the right knee and lift the torso to an upright position. You can also open the extended leg to the outer right side of the body, keeping the chest lifted and expanded.

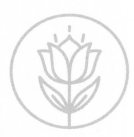

Arugula and Sweet Corn Salad

4 EARS CORN, RAW OR LIGHTLY GRILLED, CHILLED
4 OUNCES ARUGULA
1/2 RED ONION, CHOPPED
BALSAMIC VINEGAR
OLIVE OIL

Scrape the corn from the cob and mix with the arugula and onion. Sprinkle with olive oil and balsamic vinegar. Serves 4.

The Practice: Arugula and sweet corn are glorious opposites that come together to create a perfect blend for a memorable salad. Yoga means the union of opposites, like strength and stretching. The battle between two sides, that appear to be opposites, come together in one space. Seeing the oneness in each other, they found peace. "Stretch vs. Strength, God vs. Man" themes but the reality is there all the same. Triangle pose is the perfect blend of strength and stretch. While one side of the body is stretching, the other side uses strength to maintain the pose. This pose strengthens the legs as you stretch the torso. The practice is to recognize the part of you, the mind, that must stretch and expand and grow to a new consciousness, while another part of you, the faith, must stay anchored and strong during the growth period.

Triangle Pose (Trikonasana) Instruction: From Warrior 2 pose, open the front of the body while reaching to the front of the room and begin to hinge from the side, reaching to the floor. Option is to reach to the calf, foot, floor, or yoga block, and reach the opposite arm to the sky, while looking up to the extended arm.

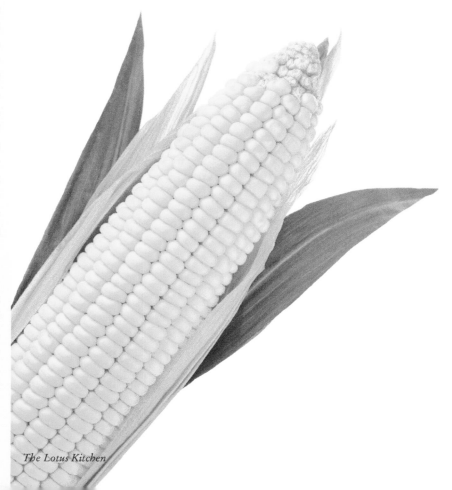

The Lotus Kitchen

Sides and Starters

For years vegetarians dining out made do with starter or side offerings, crafting a plate to satisfy the palate and nourish the body. Today, many vegetarian sides stand on their own as main dishes. Sides are meant to complement the entrée, bringing texture and flavor to the plate. Starters are great for a more expanded dining experience and many of these would be ideal for gatherings where you want to sate, not stuff your guests. And here's a Lotus Kitchen shortcut if time is pressing: sauté any seasonal vegetable in olive oil with ginger, garlic and sea salt and you have a perfect side dish or starter.

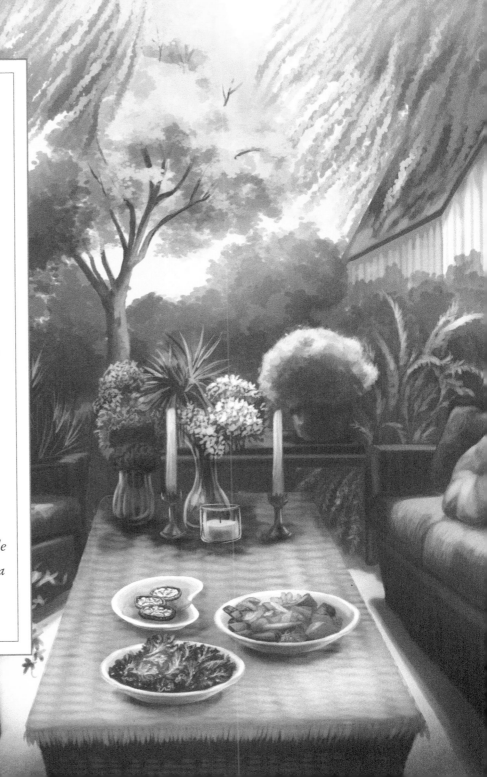

The Practice: Like the Fresh Spring Roll creation, there are many unique parts of the body temple. In yoga we begin our practice by becoming aware of our body temple. We gently awaken our body as we invite all parts of self to participate in and benefit from the experience. Ginger, citrus, soy and cilantro all subtly awaken the palate while the peppers startle with power. There are over 1,400 varieties of ginger and its healing properties are legendary. Welcome ginger to quiet rumbly stomachs, thwart a summer cold or even ease the discomfort of osteo-arthritis. Red peppers are high in vitamin A and stimulate circulation.

Mind Awareness Meditation Instruction: The body awareness meditation can be done two ways: 1. In a seated or standing position connect your mind and thoughts to one body part. As you think about the body part, breathe deeply and become aware of how it feels. Send thoughts of heal-ing and loving energy to that particular area and continue until the body is feeling whole and complete. 2. The meditation can also be done by taking a moment to contract or squeeze each body part, starting with the hands, moving up the arms and then mov-ing to the thighs and legs, repeating until the body is alive and awake. Like the first option, empowering thought and mantras, along with breathing, will enhance the med-itative practice.

Fresh Spring Rolls

8 SHEETS RICE PAPER (6-INCH ROUNDS)
1 BUNCH CILANTRO
32 BASIL LEAVES
1 RED PEPPER, THINLY SLICED
1 BUNCH GREEN ONIONS, THINLY SLICED
2 CARROTS, THINLY SLICED TO LONG RIBBONS
16 OUNCES COOKED TOFU, THINLY SLICED
1 SMALL HEAD RED CABBAGE, THINLY SLICED TO LONG RIBBONS
1/2 CUP PEANUTS, CHOPPED

Arrange equal amounts of tofu and vegetables in 8 separate piles. You will follow this procedure with each of the 8 wraps. Moisten the rice paper either by brushing a thin layer of water or simply sprinkling a little water with your fingers. The key is to make the stiff rice paper more malleable. Place the cilantro and basil leaves in the center of the circle. Add the cabbage, red pepper, green onion, carrots and tofu. Sprinkle the chopped peanuts over the vegetables. Fold rice paper in half, then fold over the sides and roll tightly from the bottom up. Slice the roll in half on the diagonal and serve with peanut sauce. Serves 8.

Peanut Sauce

2 CUPS CRUNCHY PEANUT BUTTER
1/2 CUP FRESH LIME JUICE
1/2 CUP FRESH ORANGE JUICE
1/4 CUP SOY SAUCE
1/2 CUP RICE VINEGAR
3 TABLESPOONS CRUSHED RED PEPPER
2 INCHES FRESH GINGER, PEELED AND CHOPPED
5 CLOVES GARLIC
1/2 CUP FRESH CILANTRO

Mince the garlic and ginger. In the bowl of a food processor fitted with a steel blade add the rest of the ingredients and blend until smooth. You can add less pepper if you are shy about the kick. Taste the sauce and add more soy and peppers to suit your taste. Add more orange juice for desired consistency. Add the fresh cilantro just before serving. You can either serve it warm or at room temperature.

Vegetarian Moon in the 7th House Rolls

1 TABLESPOON OLIVE OIL

1 TEASPOON SESAME OIL

1 CUP CARROTS, SHREDDED

1 EACH RED AND YELLOW BELL
  PEPPERS, SLICED

1 1/2 CUPS SNOW PEAS, THINLY
  SLICED

1 CUP GREEN CABBAGE, SHREDDED

1 CUP KALE, CHOPPED

2 CLOVES GARLIC, MINCED

1 TEASPOON FRESH GINGER, MINCED

1/4 CUP FRESH CILANTRO, DE-
  STEMMED

2 TEASPOONS SAKE

2 TEASPOONS WHITE WINE VINEGAR

1/4 CUP VEGETARIAN HOISIN SAUCE

1 TABLESPOON CHILI SAUCE

1 PACKAGE POT STICKER WRAPPERS

1 EGG, BEATEN

PEANUT OR SUNFLOWER OIL FOR
  FRYING

Heat wok (or stock pot if you are wokless) over high heat until very hot. Add oil, then garlic and ginger. Cook for a minute and then add the vegetables and cook about 6 minutes more, stirring frequently. Transfer to a bowl and add sake, rice vinegar and hoisin sauce, chili sauce and cilantro.

To make Moon Rolls, place 2 to 3 tablespoons of vegetable filling in the center of the wrapper. Using your fingers or a pastry brush spread egg all around the edges. Fold in half and pinch the edges tightly. They will resemble little half moons. Wipe the wok clean. Heat 3 cups peanut or sunflower oil on high heat. Drop egg rolls in batches of 3 and cook for 1 minute, or until golden brown. Remove with slotted spoon, place on a cookie sheet lined with paper towel to drain oil and serve immediately with dipping sauce.

Dipping Sauce

3 CLOVES GARLIC, FINELY MINCED

1 INCH FRESH GINGER, FINELY
  MINCED

1/2 CUP APRICOT PRESERVES

1/2 CUP RASPBERRY PRESERVES

4 TABLESPOONS RICE VINEGAR
  (AND/OR SAKE)

In a small bowl whisk together until smooth.

Serve with: Chinese hot mustard

Everyone can create their own dipping sauce by blending the two.

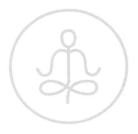

The Practice: Sun Salutation is used to heat the body. This dish warms you up inside with the heat and flavor of the ginger, garlic, and mustard. The Sun Salutation is designed to pay homage to the sun that heats the planet, and to activate our own internal sun from within. Hot mustard is a natural decongestant, aids in circulation and helps restore bacterial balance.

Sun Salutation (Suryanamaskara) Instruction: Stand at the front of your mat beginning in Mountain pose. Inhale; raise your arms above the head. Exhale, and hang from the hips to a forward bend. Inhale and lift the chest halfway. Step back into plank position. Exhale and lower the body to the mat in a push-up. Inhale to Upward-Facing Dog pose. Exhale, and push the body back to a Downward-Facing Dog pose. Inhale and lift the heels, then exhale bending the knees, and step or hop forward with both feet. Inhale the chest halfway up. Exhale and release the chest to the legs. Inhale the upper body to a standing position, and exhale the arms to Mountain, the first pose. During the Sun Salutation, visualize the sun heating your body from the inside out. Also notice that each pose will move you in a complete 360° circle.

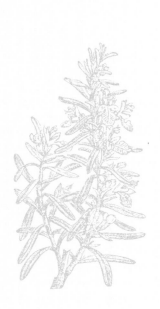

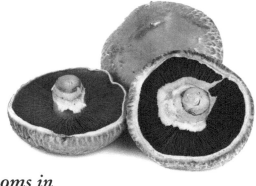

Portobello Mushrooms in Reduced Dark Cherry Balsamic Vinegar

6 Portobello mushrooms
Olive oil for brushing

Brush mushrooms with olive oil. Place on grill and weight down with a press or the flat side of a skillet. Cook about 7 minutes and flip and finish cooking for about 5 minutes. Remove from heat and cover.

Reduced Dark Cherry Balsamic Vinegar

1 cup Lucini Dark Cherry (or Fig) Balsamic
3 tablespoons butter, separated into 1-tablespoon chunks
1/4 cup flour
6 teaspoons rosemary, chopped
6 tablespoons tomatoes, chopped

In a skillet bring dark cherry balsamic to a boil. Let reduce a bit for about 3 minutes. Using a fork, stab the first tablespoon of butter and drench in the flour. Whisk into the reduced dark cherry balsamic vinegar. Repeat with the last 2 tablespoons of butter and you will have the perfect consistency. Serves 6.

To assemble:

Place one mushroom on each of 6 small plates. Pour sauce over each one. Garnish each plate with 1 teaspoon rosemary and 1 tablespoon tomatoes. Serve immediately. Also makes a wonderful sandwich.

The Practice: Like mushrooms that grow around trees, this pose profoundly grounds you to the earth. And the toes of the standing leg connect to the ground, like the roots of a tree connect it to the earth. During the practice of Tree pose visualize your feet anchored into "Mother Earth" and your body temple expanding like a tree.

Tree Pose with Om Mudra (Vrksasana) Instruction: Root firmly the standing leg into the mat and spread the toes widely. Raise the opposite leg to ankle, right below the knee, or above the knee. Extending the arms out to the side with a 45-degree bend in the elbows, bring the index fingers and thumb together to create the hand symbol of Om.

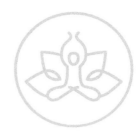

Stir-Fry Kale

Kale has become a go-to green. We eat it raw, in salads, stir-fried and in flavorful soups and stews. We even bake it to make kale chips. Kale is low in calories, high in fiber and has zero fat. Full of vitamins and calcium, kale is also a powerful antioxidant, anti-inflammatory and supports cardiovascular health.

2 TABLESPOONS OLIVE OIL

I LARGE RED ONION, CHOPPED

I LARGE GARLIC CLOVE, CHOPPED

I YELLOW PEPPER, CHOPPED

I SPRIG ROSEMARY, CHOPPED

1/2 TABLESPOON SEA SALT

1/2 CUP BASIL, CHOPPED

1/2 CUP CILANTRO, CHOPPED

I TEASPOON RED PEPPER FLAKES

1/2 CUP RAW ALMONDS

2 HEADS FRESH KALE, CHOPPED

In a wok, heat olive oil and then add the onions. Caramelize for about 10 minutes until golden brown. Add the garlic and yellow bell pepper and continue cooking until tender, about 3 minutes longer. Add the rosemary and kale and stir-fry for 1 minute. Do not overcook; the kale should be crunchy and bright green. Season to taste with red pepper and sea salt. Top with basil, cilantro and almonds. Serves 4.

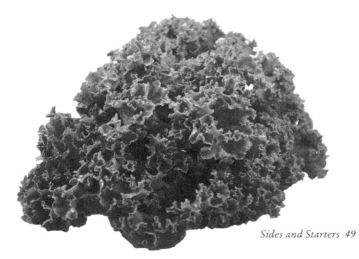

The Practice: It takes practice to master the skill of stir-frying. It appears to be a fairly simple way to prepare food, but can be challenging to get it right. It's easy to overcook vegetables, and on top of that each vegetable requires different cooking times. With practice, you'll master the art of wok cooking. Patience will guide your willing hand. "The Action of Yoga" — the action is the release of the fight, and to embrace the passion for knowledge. A simple pose like Chair pose takes hours of practice to master, and when we finally do master the pose we realize there is always something else to master within our self. The pose is but a tool.

Chair Pose (Utkatasana Fierce) Instruction: Stand tall on your mat and spread the legs hip-distance apart, while anchoring your feet by spreading your toes. Sit your hips back like you are sitting in a chair. Reach your arms long toward the sky and lengthen the torso diagonally while spreading the hands. Look toward the hand and contemplate awareness of the body. The work is to make peace with the body, asking for knowledge. "What am I to learn from this pose?"

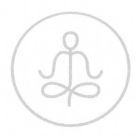

Stir-Fry Mustard and Collard Greens

1 POUND COLLARD GREENS, CHOPPED
1 POUND MUSTARD GREENS, CHOPPED
1 LARGE WHITE ONION, CHOPPED
4 LARGE SHALLOTS, MINCED
2 GARLIC CLOVES, MINCED
1 LARGE GREEN PEPPER, CHOPPED
1 TABLESPOON FRESH OREGANO
1 TABLESPOON FRESH BASIL
1 TABLESPOON FRESH THYME
1 TEASPOON YELLOW CURRY POWDER
1/2 TEASPOON WHOLE PEPPERCORN (WHOLE)
SEA SALT TO TASTE

In a large frying pan or wok sauté onions, green pepper, shallots and garlic in olive oil until tender. Add the oregano, basil, thyme, curry, peppercorn and sea salt. Stir for a minute to incorporate the flavors. Add the greens and cook until tender. (No more than 3 minutes.) Serve immediately. Serves 4 to 6.

The Practice: The stir-fry process is an amazing representation of what happens during the yoga practice. It is the heating of the veggies that releases the hidden taste and aromas within the veggies and the spices. We are preparing the food for the meditation of eating. Meditation is another word for awareness. Hatha Yoga is a practice of physical postures, or asanas, whose higher purpose is to purify the body and to prepare the body to sit in stillness during meditation. The journey is to be present with each aroma that presents itself to you. Be aware of all the tastes that come alive while eating. By now you know profoundly that yoga and eating are both practices of awareness.

Downward-Facing Dog is revisited because it is the perfect pose for the practice of awareness.

Downward-Facing Dog Pose (Adho Mukha Svanasana) Instruction: Place hands and feet on the mat and lift the hips toward the sky to create the perfect upside down V shape. Hand should be shoulder-width apart and feet hip-width apart, spreading fingers and toes to create a strong base. While practicing Downward-Facing Dog create a mantra or chant that states you are whole and renewed.

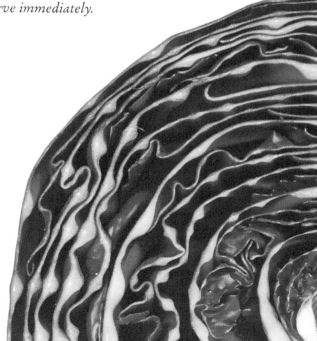

Red and Napa Cabbage Sauté

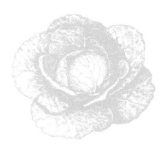

3 CLOVES GARLIC, MINCED
I RED PEPPER, SLICED
I RED ONION, SLICED
2 CUPS RED CABBAGE, SLICED
2 CUPS NAPA CABBAGE, SLICED
I CUP RAW CASHEWS, CHOPPED
SEA SALT AND CAYENNE PEPPER TO TASTE

In a large frying pan or wok, sauté the garlic and onions until tender. Add the red peppers and sauté a few minutes longer. Add the cabbage; stir for 3 minutes — no longer. Remove from heat immediately and stir in the sea salt and cayenne pepper. Place on serving platter and sprinkle with cashews. Serves 4.

The Practice: Mantra Yoga — The practice of repeating spiritual principles and divine quality to anchor our consciousness into the One Mind of God. A great pose, that requires a mantra of "Yes I Can," is Eagle Pose. Eagle is one of the most challenging poses to practice. The practice is done while cooking this dish or practicing Eagle. You will create a mantra that activates the energy of "Yes." And cabbage is a cool season crop with healing properties and vitamins that allow you to soar. Its high Vitamin K properties are especially nourishing for bone health.

Eagle Pose (Garudasana) Instruction: Stand tall on the mat and extend both arms to reach to the sides of the room. Bring both arms in front of you until the right elbow is under the left continuing to wrap the arms around each other, joining the arms into the Namaste position. Sit back into Chair pose; option is to place the right knee over the left knee balancing on one leg. Option 2: wrap the ankle around the left calf. After five breaths, release the pose and contemplate the energy of the body. Then repeat on the other side.

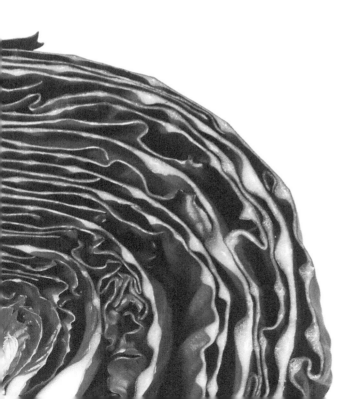

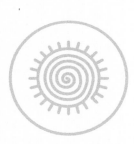

Baked Baby Yams

Baby yams are the young, edible roots of the same plant that produces fully grown yams. The coloring of baby yams can range from deep yellow to orange flesh, while the skin on the outside is usually a pale salmon color and smooth to the touch. They have a slightly more intense flavor than the more mature yam and are in season fall and winter. If they are out of season and you cannot find them you can substitute with any yam or sweet potato by simply slicing them in quarters.

3 POUNDS BABY YAMS, WASHED AND SLICED IN HALF
FRESH ROSEMARY
1/2 CUP COCONUT OIL, MELTED
SEA SALT
CAYENNE PEPPER
FRESH GARLIC

Cover the yams in coconut oil. Season with garlic, sea salt, cayenne pepper and let sit for 1 hour. Preheat oven to 350°F and bake for 1 hour or until yams are soft. Serves 4.

The Practice: When seasoned yams begin to bake, they release an aroma that can only be described as heavenly. Bhakti Yoga is the dedication and devotion in seeing the Divine within all things. Even a yam. The practice is to recognize the preparation, participation, and partaking of the meal as all-divine and good. Yoga has three parts: the preparation to do the pose, the participation of the pose itself, and the partaking of the benefits of the pose. One of the poses is the Seated Staff Pose. As we sit, we begin the preparation by raising our arms and that energy takes us into the pose. During the pose we dig deep within to find the strength, and once it is over, there is a "Wow" sensation.

Staff Pose (Dandasana) Instruction: From a seated position, straighten legs, flexing the balls of the feet and heels, and spreading the toes. Place hands flat on the floor next to the hips with palms down. Lengthen the spine and continue to lift the top of the head, with the chin three inches away from the chest. Support your natural spine, gazing forward.

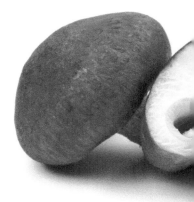

Sautéed Spinach and Shiitake Mushrooms

I LARGE RED ONION, CHOPPED
I LARGE GARLIC CLOVE, CHOPPED
I SPRIG ROSEMARY, CHOPPED
I/2 TEASPOON SEA SALT
I/4 TEASPOON CHINESE FIVE-SPICE
I POUND OF SPINACH, BAGGED OR DE-LEAFED
2 CUPS OF WHOLE SHIITAKE MUSHROOMS

Sauté onion and garlic until tender. Add shiitake mushrooms and continue sautéing until the mushrooms are tender. Add spinach for 1 minute. Do not overcook; keep crunchy and bright green. Season with five-spice, sea salt and rosemary. Serves 4.

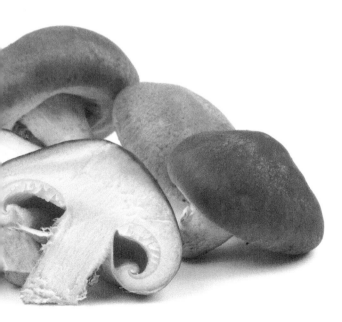

The Practice: Like yoga, spinach is a natural cleanser of the body. Both can help heal the digestive system, cleanse the colon, and detoxify the body. One of the principles of yoga is Shucha or Purity. Yoga is the deepest way to detoxify the body. As you begin your practice, set the intentions that the body temple will release all things that do not serve it any longer. As you begin to eat the spinach, know that the power of this green leafy delight balances the mind, body, and spirit. One way to stimulate detoxification during yoga is the Sun Salutation.

Sun Salutation (Suryanamaskara) Instruction: Stand at the front of your mat beginning in Mountain pose. Inhale and raise your arms above the head. Exhale and hang from the hips to a forward bend. Inhale and lift the chest halfway. Step back into plank position. Exhale and lower the body to the mat in a push-up. Inhale to Upward-Facing Dog pose. Exhale and push the body to a Downward-Facing Dog pose. Inhale and lift the heels, then exhale bending the knees and step or hop forward with both feet. Inhale the chest halfway up. Exhale and release the chest to the legs. Inhale the upper body to a standing position then exhale the arms to Mountain, the first pose. Visualize the sun healing your body from the inside out.

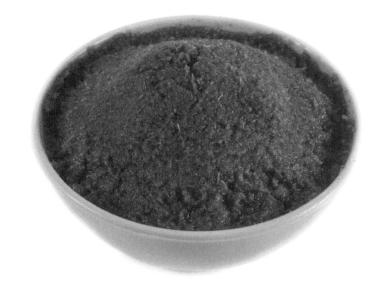

The Practice: Coconut milk is the milk of contentment; the milk of love. In Yoga, Santosha is the principle of contentment. Like the physical practice you have said yes to, be accepting of yourself as you eat this meal. The practice is to be content in any situation. When the highway of life is bumpy, make the decision to be content by sipping the nectar of the island Gods.

Cow Face Pose (Gomukhasana) Instruction: Starting in a seated position, place the bent right knee on top of the bent left knee perfectly stacked. Feel the opening of the knee joint settling into the pose. Bring your left arm up to the sky and bend the left arm behind the head and the neck pointing downward, resting the palm on the upper back. Bring the right arm to the side, bend the right elbow and move the right hand behind your back with your finger going upward. Try to bring the fingers together to create a bond. If you cannot reach, use your T-shirt or a towel to create the connection. Mentally think about opening the front of the body. Allow the awareness of the flexibility of the triceps, shoulders and hips. This pose will reveal all.

Assorted Seasonal Vegetables with Green Curry

3 TABLESPOONS OLIVE OIL

2 TABLESPOONS GREEN CURRY PASTE

1 1/2 POUNDS ASSORTED VEGETABLES (CARROTS, ZUCCHINI, GREEN BEANS, EGGPLANT, PEPPERS, WINTER SQUASH)

4 KAFFIR LIME LEAVES

2 LEMONGRASS STALKS, BRUISED AND CUT

2 CUPS UNSWEETENED COCONUT MILK

1/2 POUND SNOW PEAS

15 BASIL LEAVES

You can use any assorted vegetables that you like. Chop them in a similar size, about one-inch chunks. In a wok or frying pan heat the oil. Add the green curry paste and stir-fry until bubbly and fragrant. Add the vegetables, kaffir lime leaves and lemongrass. Cook until the vegetables are soft. Add the snow peas and cook for another minute. Stir in the coconut milk and bring to a gentle boil. Simmer and stir occasionally for 5 minutes. Stir in the basil and serve over rice.

Garlic Minty Roasted Potatoes

16 POTATOES (WE LIKE A COMBINATION OF WHITE, RED, PURPLE, FINGERLING,
    YAMS AND SWEET POTATOES, DEPENDING ON WHAT IS AVAILABLE)
1/2 CUP OLIVE OIL
KOSHER SALT, TO TASTE
FRESHLY GROUND BLACK PEPPER
8 GARLIC CLOVES, FINELY CHOPPED
1/4 CUP FRESH MINT LEAVES, COARSELY CHOPPED

Preheat oven to 350°F. Prick the potatoes with the tines of a fork and arrange them on a baking sheet. Bake for 1 1/2 hours. Cut the potatoes into quarters and place them in a serving bowl. While they are still hot, toss them with the oil, salt, pepper and garlic. Gently toss in the mint. This twist on a potato salad can be served warm or at room temperature. Serves 8.

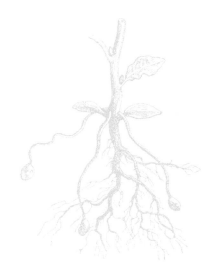

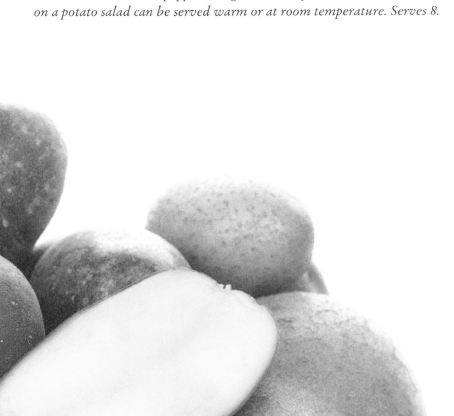

The Practice: Potatoes are regarded as one of the brain foods, considered to help memory and to stimulate brain cells. Swadhyaya, the yoga principle of Self-Education, is the quest for knowledge. What a great combination. The practice while creating this dish is to know that all situations are an opportunity to expand your consciousness. Every situation is a learning situation. The Easy Pose (Sukhasana) is the posture that we surrender our self to while learning the experience of yoga.

The Easy Pose Meditation Instruction: Sitting with your buttocks on the mat, cross your legs with your ankles under your thighs. Rest your hands on your knees, press both hips toward the floor and close your eyes, and breathe. Allow your thoughts to open to knowledge and learning. Set the intention to know more as you practice.

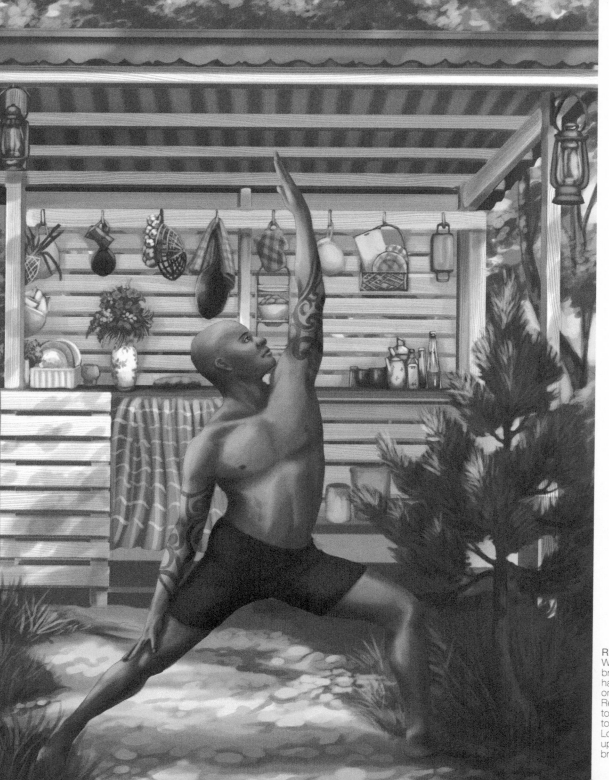

REVERSE WARRIOR
With the knee bent,
bring the opposing
hand down to rest
on the extended leg.
Reach the other arm up
towards the ceiling and
to the back of the room.
Look straight ahead or
up at the ceiling and
breathe.

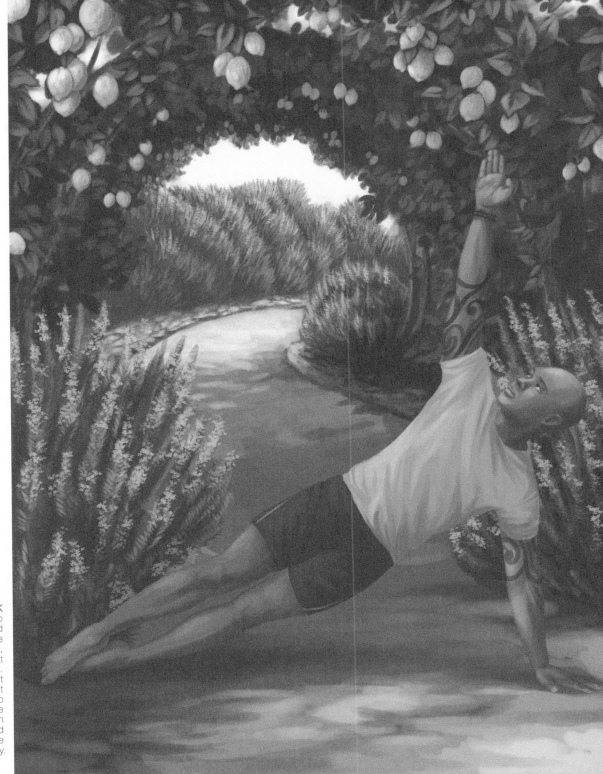

SIDE PLANK
Place left hand on to the mat, rotate and shift onto the outside edge of your left foot, and stack your right foot on top of the left. Now swing your right hand onto your right hip, turn your torso to the right support the weight of your body on the outer left foot and left hand. Reach the right arm to the sky.

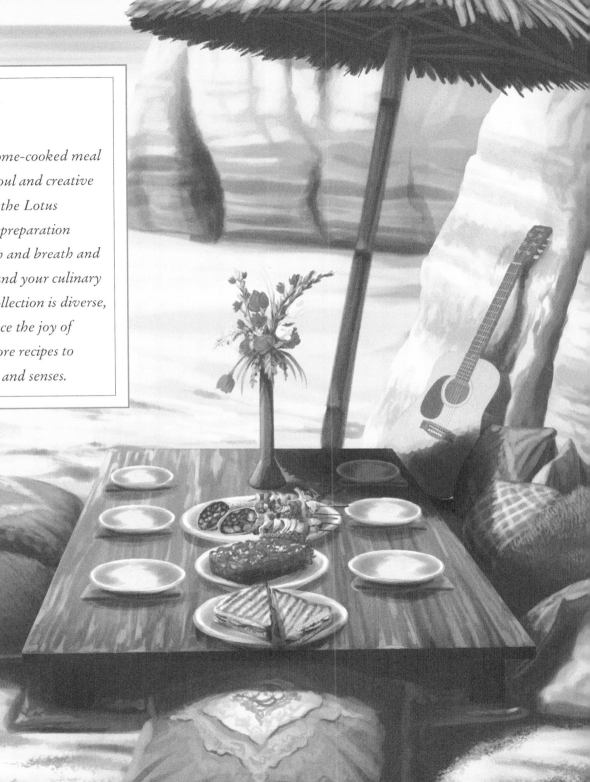

Entrées

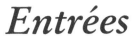

The entrée of any home-cooked meal reflects your heart, soul and creative spirit on a plate. For the Lotus Kitchen chef, entrée preparation incorporates strength and breath and a willingness to expand your culinary reach. This entrée collection is diverse, not complex. Embrace the joy of creation as you explore recipes to ignite the taste buds and senses.

Jambalaya

The Practice: When we think of Jambalaya, the sensation is heat. Heat is the great detoxifier used for healing. One of the yoga meditations for breathing expertise is called the "Breath of Fire." The practice is used to generate heat and increases your level of energy by activating the energy flow in your body, quickly oxygenating your blood, thus helping the body detoxify itself. The practice is to recognize both the dish and the "Breath of Fire" having the same ability for healing.

The Breath of Fire Instruction Option #1 — The Vinyasa Practice: Sit on your yoga mat and place your right hand on your stomach. Take a few seconds and center yourself. Inhale through your nose and push outward as you inhale, keeping the mouth closed. One can create a large amount of heat, your own "Breath of Fire." (Should not be done during pregnancy or menstruation.) Option #2 — The Kundalini Practice: From kneeling, sit back onto the heels and raise arms over your head with a wide distance from hand to hand, creating a "V"-like shape. Squeeze the four fingers into the hand with the thumbs extended upward. This will activate energy throughout the chakra system. Open the mouth and lay the tongue over the bottom lip and begin to pant like a puppy dog, with an even pace between inhales and exhales. Once this technique is learned, practice Breath of Fire with a closed mouth.

2 CUPS COOKED BROWN OR BASMATI RICE
2 CUPS COOKED PINTO BEANS
2 CUPS COOKED WHITE BEANS
2 CUPS COOKED BLACK BEANS
1 MEDIUM ONION, CHOPPED
1/4 CUP ROASTED GARLIC, CHOPPED
1 MEDIUM RED PEPPER, CHOPPED
1 CUP CHOPPED SWEET CHERRY TOMATOES

5 CUPS ASSORTED VEGETABLES — CAULIFLOWER, BROCCOLI, GREEN BEANS, CARROTS (ANYTHING IN SEASON)
1/2 CUP CILANTRO
1/2 CUP BASIL
1/3 CUP ROSEMARY
1 CUP RED OR YELLOW CURRY SAUCE
1 CUP SWEET CHILI SAUCE
CAYENNE PEPPER
SEA SALT

In a large pot sauté the onions, garlic and red pepper. Add tomatoes and assorted vegetables and beans. Add seasoning and sauces. Bring to a boil and let simmer for 2 hours. Add beans and rice. Serves 8.

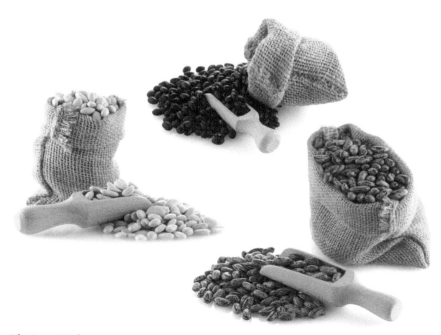

Baked Spinach Cakes

These special cakes were created for a cooking segment and were a big hit with the crew. They can also be served as an appetizer and are equally delicious the next day. It's imperative that the spinach is well drained to avoid a runny cake.

16 OUNCES FRESH SPINACH (1 BAG OR 1 LARGE BUNCH), WASHED WELL AND CHOPPED FINE OR
16 OUNCES FROZEN SPINACH, THAWED AND WELL SQUEEZED, DRAINED OF AS MUCH LIQUID AS POSSIBLE
1 CUP PART-SKIM RICOTTA CHEESE
1/2 CUP FINELY SHREDDED PARMESAN CHEESE, PLUS MORE FOR GARNISH
2 LARGE EGGS, BEATEN
3 CLOVES GARLIC, MINCED
1/2 TEASPOON FRESHLY GRATED NUTMEG
SALT AND FRESHLY GROUND PEPPER TO TASTE

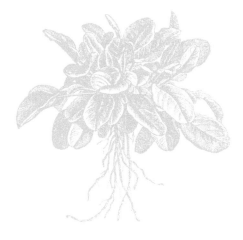

Preheat oven to 400°F. In a medium bowl add spinach, ricotta, Parmesan, eggs, garlic, nutmeg, salt and pepper; stir to combine. Coat a 12-cup standard-size muffin pan with cooking spray. Divide the spinach mixture among the 12 cups; they will be very full and very dense. Sprinkle with Parmesan cheese. Bake the spinach cakes until set, about 30 minutes. Let stand in the pan for 5 minutes. Loosen the edges with a knife and place on a large serving platter. Serve warm or at room temperature with a dollop of sour cream or almond yogurt. Serves 6.

The Practice: The Sat Nam "Truth is my reality" — Sat Nam is a mantra commonly used in Kundalini Yoga and amongst its practitioners. It is frequently repeated three times at the end of a yoga session. But the importance of Sat Nam is the meaning. Sat Nam has been interpreted as: Truth is my identity, truth is my reality, and truth is my authentic self. The mantra is also a recognition that God, goodness, or truth is in all things and heaven is present in this very moment. The practice is to recognize truth in every bite of the baked spinach pie. Goodness and love is the truth of everything. Sat Nam can be used in every pose to remind you of the truth as a way to focus the mind before meditation.

Unity Collard Green Wraps

The Practice: Yoga is the pathway to the realization of your oneness with your higher self and everyone else's as there is no separation. The yoking of the class is the mental and spiritual yoga practice that happens during each group session. The realization that we are all one is the practice of unification. As you eat the Unity Collard Green Wrap, recognize your oneness with everything. Know the power of unity with all things. In your yoga practice or class, see all the examples of yoke: instructor yokes to students, student yoke to each other. The mind is one with the body during the pose. Downward-Facing Dog is the perfect pose of oneness and students come back to Down Dog many times during the practice. As you find your way through *The Lotus Kitchen*, continue to master your Down Dog and be mindful that many students, all over the world, are doing the pose simultaneously. That is a beautiful expression of unity.

Downward-Facing Dog Pose (Adho Mukha Svanasana) Instruction: Place hands and feet on the mat and lift the hips toward the sky to create the perfect upside down V shape. Hands should be shoulder-width apart and feet hip-width apart, spreading fingers and toes to create a strong base. While practicing Downward-Facing Dog, create a mantra or chant that states you are whole and renewed.

Aside from being playful and flavorful this recipe rests on a comfortable perch atop the good-for-you department. Ginger and garlic are long known for their healing properties. Peppers contribute to cardiovascular health. Basil delivers antibacterial and anti-inflammatory properties while the lemongrass doubles as anti-inflammatory and antioxidant. Meanwhile cilantro contains essential oils that help with digestion, and is an analgesic and aphrodisiac. On top of that? They're really really tasty.

2 TABLESPOONS GARLIC PASTE	2 CUPS BASIL, CHOPPED
2 TABLESPOONS GINGER PASTE	2 CUPS MINT, CHOPPED
2 TABLESPOONS LEMONGRASS PASTE	2 CUPS GREEN ONION, CHOPPED
3 CUPS FIRM TOFU	3 CUPS RAW PEANUTS, SLIVERED
1 SMALL YELLOW ONION, DICED	3 CUPS CARROTS, SLIVERED
1 RED PEPPER, CHOPPED	3 CUPS ARUGULA, CHOPPED
6 TEASPOONS OLIVE OIL	3 CUPS ALFALFA SPROUTS
2 CUPS CILANTRO, CHOPPED	6 COLLARD LEAVES, WHOLE

Mix together the ginger, garlic and lemongrass pastes. In a small frying pan sauté the onion and red pepper in the olive oil. When tender add the tofu and sauté to coat. Let cool for a moment, then place in a food processor and blend on medium speed to form a paste. Toss together the herbs, peanuts, carrots, arugula, and alfalfa sprouts. Time to assemble these lovelies. Take a large collard green and lay it with the light side facing up. Spread the ginger, garlic and lemongrass mixture on the leaf. Add a layer of the tofu paste. Add 1 1/2 cups of the herb mixture and spread over the entire leaf. Grab the bottom of the leaf and tightly roll until wrapped. Slice in half. Serves 4.

Lentil Stew

1/2 CUP OLIVE OIL

6 CLOVES GARLIC

1 LARGE ONION, CHOPPED

3 CARROTS, CHOPPED

1 SMALL HEAD BROCCOLI, CHOPPED

1 BUNCH KALE, CHOPPED

1 BUNCH SPINACH, CLEANED AND CHOPPED

2 CUPS LITTLE GREEN LENTILS

4 CUPS VEGETABLE STOCK

6 CUPS MARINARA SAUCE

1/2 CUP RED WINE

SALT AND PEPPER TO TASTE

2 TABLESPOONS BASIL

2 TABLESPOONS THYME

In a large soup pot, heat oil over medium heat. Add onions and garlic and sauté. Add lentils, carrots, broccoli, kale and spinach and give a quick sauté. Add the rest of the ingredients and cook over low heat for about 1 hour. Serves 8.

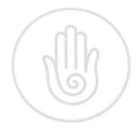

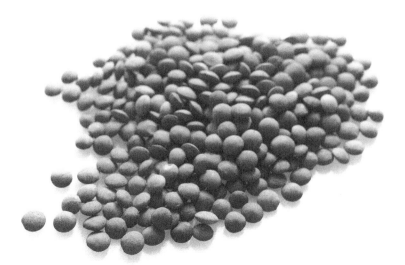

The Practice: Lentils come from India, the home of yoga practice. In India, deep practice is to see the Universe working in all things. In the yoga practice it is called Ishvara-Pranidhana, which means dedication to the Divine or the Power of Surrender. The practice is to see the Divine in every lentil. Take the time to feel each legume and bless it. See the presence of life within each lentil. See how each one is different, but is also the same. The pea is the representation of the work and its inhabitance.

Breathing Meditation Instruction: Sit in a comfortable position. Relax and place the hands lightly on the knees. Close the eyes and begin to breathe. Be especially mindful of when you inhale and when you exhale. Begin to count each breath, and as you breathe create a mantra that incorporates your intention. For example: "I breathe this breath for the preparation of this meal." "I am aware of the Universe." "This food and I are one." "I surrender to the peace." "I surrender to the experience."

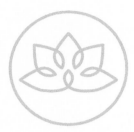

Roasted Veggie Panini

1 RED ONION, SLICED	SEA SALT AND PEPPER TO TASTE
2 RED PEPPERS, HALVED	2 LARGE VERY RIPE AVOCADOS
2 GREEN PEPPERS, HALVED	2 CUPS ALFALFA SPROUTS
2 YELLOW PEPPERS, HALVED	8 SLICES MULTIGRAIN OR PITA
1 EGGPLANT, SLICED IN ROUNDS	BREAD
3 CLOVES GARLIC, MINCED	2 TABLESPOONS OLIVE OIL FOR
3 TABLESPOONS OLIVE OIL	COATING PAN

To roast the vegetables: *Gently toss the garlic, onions, peppers and eggplant in olive oil. Season with sea salt and pepper. Place vegetables in a roasting pan in a single layer. Roast for 45 minutes in a preheated oven.*

To assemble: *Spread avocado on each slice of bread. Place 2 slices of onion, 1 each of the halved peppers and 1 eggplant round on bread. Add 1/2 cup alfalfa sprouts. Close the sandwich and give it a good press.*

To Panini: *Have a large and slightly smaller skillet ready. Place the large skillet over medium heat. Coat the pan with a half-tablespoon of olive oil. Place the panini in the pan and press down with the bottom of the smaller pan. Once golden brown, flip the sandwich and place the bottom of the smaller pan over it. When it is golden brown, remove from pan, cut in half and serve. Continue with the other 3 sandwiches. Serves 4.*

The Practice: The Veggie Panini is the perfect example of yoga: all the goodness of the practice is sandwiched between two physical anchoring points, the warm-up/sun salutation, and the final corpse pose. Poses are always practiced starting with intentions and finished with achievements. The asana or pose begins with the willingness, and is finished with an insight. When beginning the pose there is always a sense of struggle until we find peace. Remember that yoga is a yoking or natural expression of bringing or connecting the many delectable pieces of goodness together into one.

Chair Pose (Utkatasana Fierce) Instruction: Stand tall on your mat and spread the legs at hip-distance apart. Anchor your feet by spreading your toes. Sit your hips back as if you are sitting in a chair. Reach your arms long toward the sky and lengthen the torso diagonally while spreading the fingers or the hands. Look toward the hand and contemplate awareness of the body.

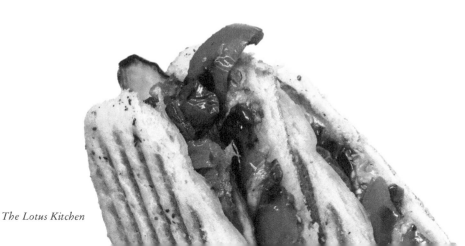

The Lotus Kitchen

Tempeh Boat

We created this dish to remind us that each meal carries blessings for our life. Skip was fooling around in the kitchen while we were playing with this recipe and said, "Look, Gwen, here is a boat full of blessings!" You can eat the tempeh filling with a fork or you can fold the cabbage and eat it like a taco.

Tempeh is a traditional soy product that comes from Indonesia but unlike tofu it is processed less. There is a natural process of fermenting the soybean to create a dense vegan product that can be used in veggie burgers, vegetarian bacon and other meat substitutions. High in vitamin B-12, it allows you to absorb all the other nutrients floating in our boat.

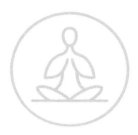

4 CUPS PREPARED TEMPEH, CHOPPED INTO 1/4-INCH CUBES	TO TASTE
1 CUP SHIITAKE MUSHROOMS, CHOPPED FINE	3 TABLESPOONS OLIVE OR COCONUT OIL
1/4 CUP CILANTRO, TO TASTE	4 RED CABBAGE LEAVES — THIS IS FOR "THE BOAT." THE LARGE OUTER LEAVES WORK BEST.
1/4 CUP BASIL	
1/4 CUP MINT	4 CUPS ARUGULA
1/2 CUP RED ONIONS, CHOPPED	1 CUP ALFALFA SPROUTS
3 CLOVES GARLIC, MINCED	1 CUP CARROT SLIVERS
PINCH OF SALT AND GROUND PEPPER	1 CUP RAW PEANUTS, FINELY CHOPPED

Heat oil in a sauté pan over medium-high heat until just smoking and then add garlic and onions and cook until tender, about 5 minutes. Add in the tempeh and the shiitake mushrooms and cook for 10 minutes, stirring constantly. Add in the herbs and salt and pepper and stir for another 5 minutes. Take off the stovetop and cover while you prepare the boats.

Place 4 red cabbage leaves (your boat) on a cutting board hollow end up. Place a bed of arugula (1 cup each) on the 4 cabbage leaves. Place 1/4 of your tempeh mixture over the arugula. Garnish with a layer of alfalfa sprouts, followed by the carrot slivers and finish with the chopped peanuts. Place each boat on a plate and serve. Serves 4.

The Practice: Navasana, also known as Boat Pose, allows us to be a vessel to carry blessings to the world. Navasana reminds us to be the tool to share the goodness of life, joy, peace, oneness, and love to all that we meet. The practice is to set the intention to be a giver of love everywhere you go. As you place the ingredients of the tofu boat into the cabbage, acknowledge yourself as the divine blessing you are. We created this dish to remind us that each meal carries blessings for our life.

Boat Pose (Navasana) Instruction: Boat pose Navasana is the pose with legs and arms extended in the air with our gaze being on the limbs. Begin seated and place the hands on the mat behind you. Extend your legs long toward the front of the room and begin to lean back, finding your tail bone. Once you are balanced, onto the lumbar spine and tail bone, bend the knees and reach your hands to the sky. Option: Bring the legs off the floor into tabletop. Option 2: Extend and straighten the legs.

Slow-Cooked Red Beans and Red Lentils

1 LARGE RED ONION, CHOPPED

1 LARGE GARLIC CLOVE, CHOPPED

2 LARGE SHALLOTS, CHOPPED

PEPPERCORN (CRUSHED)

CORIANDER SEEDS (WHOLE)

SEA SALT

2 CUPS RED LENTILS

2 CUPS SMALL RED BEANS

FRESH THYME

FRESH ROSEMARY

FRESH OREGANO

FRESH BASIL

3 CUPS WATER

Combine everything in the crock pot. Cook on low for 8 to 10 hours. Give it a good stir and allow it to cook a half hour before serving. Serves 4 to 6.

The Practice: The slow cooking of yoga, like the slow cooking of the lentils, is a process. The practice of cooking this dish is patience. Yoga is all about patience and holding the stillness. Sometimes we must be still until the enlightenment comes. Be patient until the stew of transformation is complete. Like this meal, if you remove the heat from the practice too soon, you can miss the miracle. When you feel you are ready to end a pose, hold it for one more breath. Be patient and have faith that the message is coming through. Like this lentil dish, it takes time for the herbs and spices to awaken to their fullness. Each pose of yoga is the same. Be still until the flavor of life is awakened from each asana.

Mountain Pose (Tadasana) Instruction: Stand tall at the top of your mat with feet hip-distance apart. Spread the toes to create a strong base. Draw the shoulders away from the ears and open the arms while spreading your fingers. Be the mountain. Inhabit its strength and grace. While standing in Mountain pose, become the mountain. What qualities of the mountain best represent you? Connect with the attributes that best describe your journey.

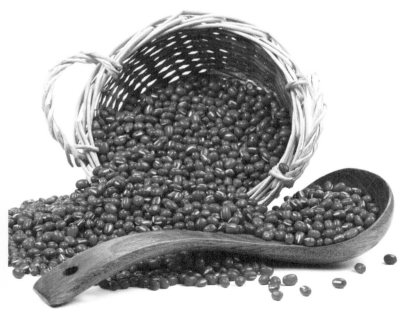

Raw Pad Thai

Many natural foods markets allow you to grind your own peanut butter. If that's not an option, find a peanut butter that is as raw as possible. Another key ingredient in this dish is the kelp noodle, made from an edible brown seaweed high in iodine. Marketed as a low-calorie alternative to pasta and other noodle varieties, kelp noodles are a staple in raw and gluten-free diets. Kelp noodles are said to improve thyroid health, help protect against osteoporosis, promote weight loss and enhance heart health. Green tea kelp noodles offer the added benefits of the powerful antioxidants found in green tea.

12-OUNCE PACKAGE KELP NOODLES OR GREEN TEA KELP NOODLES
2 CUPS MUSTARD GREENS
2 CUPS ARUGULA
10 BASIL LEAVES, CHOPPED
1/2 CUP RAW PEANUTS
1/2 CUP GREEN ONIONS

Place the kelp noodles in a large bowl and toss with the sauce. Toss the arugula and mustard greens together and place on a large serving plate. Pour the dressed noodles over the greens and garnish with basil, peanuts and green onions. Serves 2. Can easily be doubled.

Sauce:
4 TABLESPOONS PEANUT BUTTER (WHOLE FOOD OR RAW SECTION IN MARKET)
1/3 CUP COCONUT OIL
1 TABLESPOON SOY SAUCE
1/3 CUP CORIANDER SEEDS
2 WHOLE THAI CHILI PEPPERS (RED)
JUICE AND ZEST OF 1 MEDIUM LEMON
1/2 CUP WATER

Blend all ingredients in food processor until completely mixed.

The Practice: Raw food is at its freshest in the raw state. Yoga is also both raw and fresh. The rawness of yoga is about not judging yourself. No matter what or how you look, you are perfect and complete. When standing in front of a mirror, be willing to bless your divine self, even during the raw rough spots. Each day, when we practice, see the newness, and the freshness of yoga for that day. Every practice is new.

Tree Pose (Vrksasana) Instruction: Root firmly the standing leg into the mat and spread the toes widely. Raise the opposite leg to the ankle, right below the knee or just above the knee. Place arms in praying hands over the heart or directly above the head.

Vegan Burrito

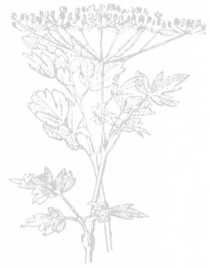

4 WHOLE GRAIN TORTILLAS
4 CUPS COOKED BLACK BEANS
4 CUPS COOKED BROWN RICE
I CUP VEGAN GUACAMOLE (RECIPE FOLLOWS)
4 TABLESPOONS SUN-DRIED TOMATO PASTE
I CUP RED PEPPERS, SLICED LENGTHWISE
I CUP YELLOW PEPPERS, SLICED LENGTHWISE
I RED ONION, SLICED LENGTHWISE
3 CLOVES GARLIC, MINCED
I JALAPEÑO, MINCED
3 TABLESPOONS OLIVE OIL
4 TABLESPOONS EACH BASIL AND CILANTRO, CHOPPED

In a sauté pan heat olive oil over medium heat until just smoking. Toss in the onions and garlic and cook until tender, about 5 minutes. Add the peppers and continue sautéing for another 5 minutes and remove from heat.

For each burrito you will lay out a tortilla and then layer in the center 1 tablespoon sun-dried tomato paste followed by 1/4 cup vegan guacamole. Then layer 1 cup beans followed by 1 cup rice. Then layer 1/4 of the pepper mixture. Then sprinkle with the fresh herbs. From the bottom of the tortilla fold the burrito in half. Fold the right and left side edges inside and roll from the bottom up to the top. Continue with the 3 remaining burritos. Makes 4.

Vegan Guacamole

2 LARGE RIPE AVOCADOS
I/4 RED ONION, MINCED
I CLOVE GARLIC, MINCED
I/4 CUP CILANTRO
I SMALL TOMATO, CHOPPED FINE

Mix together to make a paste.

The Lotus Kitchen

The Practice: The Vegan rolls are a representation of no animal harmed. The Vegan philosophy is anchored in nonviolence to any living thing. In yoga, the principle of nonviolence is called "Ahimsa." This practice not only pertains to others, but also to one's self. The practice is to be mindful of how we treat ourselves. Are we overworking? Are we eating the wrong food? How we treat ourselves affects the way we treat each other.

Corpse Pose (Savasana) Instruction: We lay on our backs in full rest, fully experiencing the pleasures of the breath and the moment.

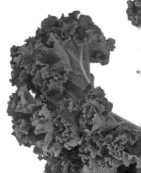

Holy Kale

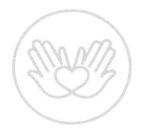

1 RED ONION, CHOPPED

3 CLOVES GARLIC, MINCED

1 RED PEPPER, CHOPPED

1 GREEN PEPPER, CHOPPED

1/2 JALAPEÑO PEPPER, MINCED

2 LARGE EGGPLANTS, CHOPPED IN CUBES

1 HEAD KALE, CHOPPED

1 PINT CHERRY TOMATOES

1/2 TEASPOON SEA SALT

ZEST OF 1 LEMON

1 TABLESPOON YELLOW CURRY POWDER

1/2 CUP CILANTRO, SLIVERED FOR GARNISH

1/2 CUP BASIL, SLIVERED FOR GARNISH

In a large frying pan or wok, sauté garlic and onions. Add the green, red and jalapeño peppers and eggplant and sauté for a few minutes. Gently add the cherry tomatoes and kale and cook 2 minutes longer. Season with the lemon zest, curry, and sea salt. Place on a serving platter and garnish with the basil and cilantro. Serves 4.

The Practice: The practice of being Holy is the path of truthfulness. Satya in Sanskrit means unchangeable or absolute truthfulness; this is a holy and righteous way of life, a way of being. As you eat the Holy Kale, contemplate your truthfulness with self. Yoga is the path to honesty and truthfulness. In *The Lotus Kitchen*, we revisit Downward-Facing Dog many times. It is the perfect recover pose during your practice. It is also the pose that most Yogis find a place of surrender and truth. It is the ultimate bowing pose, surrendering to our personal truth about our body, mind and spirit.

Downward-Facing Dog Pose (Adho Mukha Svanasana) Instruction: Place hands and feet on the mat and lift hips toward the sky to create the perfect upside down V shape. Hands should be shoulder-width apart and feet hip-width apart, spreading fingers and toes to create a strong base. While practicing Downward-Facing Dog, create a mantra or chant that states you are whole and renewed.

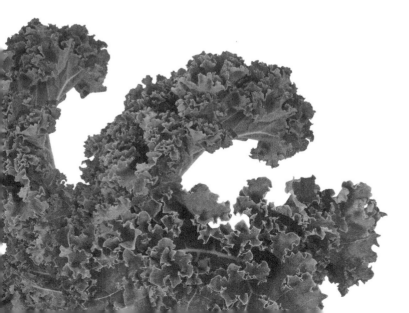

The Practice: Both the open-face sandwich and Cow Face pose (Gomukhasana) are to have a sensation of openness and freedom to show all. Like the ingredients of this culinary treat, this pose reveals the flexibility of every joint of the body, all at once.

Cow Face Pose (Gomukhasana) Instruction: Starting in a seated position, place the bent right knee on top of the bent left knee perfectly stacked. Feel the opening of the knee joints and hip joint settling into the pose. Bring your left arm up to the sky and bend the left resting the palm on the upper back. Bring the right arm to the side, bend the right elbow and move the right hand behind your back with your finger going upward. Try to bring the fingers together to create a bond. If you cannot reach, use your T-shirt or a towel to create the connection. Mentally think about opening the front of the body. Allow the awareness of the flexibility of the triceps, shoulders, and hips. This pose will reveal all.

Open-Face Hummus Sandwich

WHOLE GRAIN BAGEL, SPLIT IN HALF
FRESH HUMMUS
1/2 CUP WASHED SPINACH
1 TOMATO, SLICED

Spread hummus on each side of bagel, toasted or plain. Lay spinach on top of hummus, then place layer of tomatoes on top of the spinach. Simple and simply delicious, especially if you prepare your own hummus.

Basic Hummus

2 CUPS (COOKED OR CANNED) GARBANZO BEANS (CHICKPEAS)
3 CLOVES GARLIC, PEELED
6–8 TABLESPOONS LEMON JUICE
1 TABLESPOON SALT
1/2 CUP TAHINI (SESAME SEED BUTTER)
2 TABLESPOONS OLIVE OIL
1/4 TEASPOON CUMIN
1/4 TEASPOON CAYENNE PEPPER

Finely chop the garlic in a food processor. Add the remaining ingredients and puree until smooth, stopping twice to scrape down the sides of the bowl. Transfer to a serving bowl and serve at room temperature with vegetables and pita bread. Makes 3 cups.

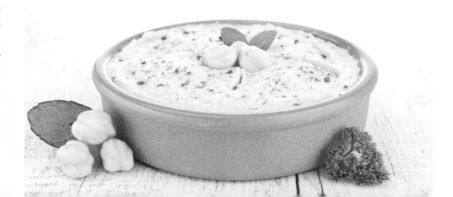

Baked Lentil Loaf with Vegetarian Country Gravy

1 BAY LEAF

3 CUPS WATER

2 CUPS LENTILS

1 SMALL RED ONION, FINELY
  CHOPPED

4 CLOVES GARLIC

1 TABLESPOON OLIVE OIL

3 CARROTS, FINELY CHOPPED

1 RED BELL PEPPER, FINELY CHOPPED

1 CUP ROLLED OATS

1 CUP WHOLE WHEAT BREAD CRUMBS

1 TABLESPOON SESAME OIL

JUICE OF 1 LEMON

1/2 TEASPOON LEMON ZEST

1 TEASPOON THYME

1 TEASPOON ROSEMARY

1/2 TEASPOON CAYENNE PEPPER

In a medium saucepan cook the lentils and the bay leaf until soft, about 45 minutes until all of the water is absorbed. Set aside. Sauté the onions and garlic in the olive oil until the onion is translucent, about 5 minutes. Add the carrots, celery, red peppers and spices and sauté about 15 minutes more. Let cool. Add veggie mixture to lentil mixture, mix well and then add oats, bread crumbs, and lemon zest and sesame oil. Mix well and pour into a greased loaf pan. Bake in a preheated oven at 350ºF for about 45 minutes until firm. Serve warm with Country Gravy. Serves 6 to 8.

Country Gravy

3 TABLESPOONS OLIVE OIL

4 PORTOBELLO MUSHROOMS, SLICED
  1/4-INCH THICK, THEN SLICED IN
  FOURTHS

1 SMALL ONION, THINLY SLICED

2 CLOVES GARLIC

2 CUPS VEGETABLE STOCK

1/2 TEASPOON THYME

1/2 TEASPOON ROSEMARY

PINCH SALT AND PEPPER

3 TABLESPOONS WHOLE WHEAT
  FLOUR OR GLUTEN-FREE FLOUR

FRESH THYME AND ROSEMARY TO
  FLOAT ON THE TOP

In a skillet, heat 1 1/2 tablespoons olive oil. Add mushrooms, garlic and onion and sauté for approximately 7 minutes until the mushrooms are cooked and the onions are translucent. Remove from skillet and set aside. Heat remaining oil and add flour and whisk until smooth and cook 30 seconds. Add stock in a steady stream while continuing to whisk and cook for 5 minutes. Stir in reserve mushrooms, thyme and rosemary and cook 5 minutes more. Season with salt and pepper.

The Practice: This recipe requires a baking ceremony. Vipassana Meditation, which means to see things as they really are, is one of India's most ancient techniques of meditation. This is a ceremony of long extended stillness in one pose, sometimes in discomfort, in a spiritual oven, and baking until you receive an insight or until you are done. This is the meditation that allows one to see how strong they really are. The principle behind this breathing practice is overcoming obstacles. If one can overcome the discomfort of this meditation session, you can overcome any obstacles of life. Lotus Pose or Seated Relaxation Pose is used in this long practice of sitting and meditation.

Lotus Pose or Seated Relaxation Pose (Padmasana) Instruction: Lotus pose or Seated Relaxation Pose can be done gentle or deep. Sit on the mat with legs crossed for a gentle pose for the hips. Option: cross ankle across the opposite hip, crossing the other leg and ankle on top of the opposite leg, reaching to the opposite hip. There are two hand positions that can be used, "Metta" which means loving kindness, or "Buddha Mudra," which promotes fine-tuning of the mind and activates relaxation of the body. "Metta" hand position: lay hands lightly on the knees in the hand position, palms open, facing the sky, with eyes closed. In the Buddha Mudra hand position, your right hand is facing up with the first finger and thumb together, and the left hand pointing downward, fingertips touching the mat, palm facing the knee.

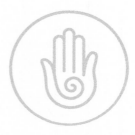

Stuffed Zucchini

4 MEDIUM ZUCCHINI, HALVED LENGTHWISE

1 TABLESPOON OLIVE OIL

1 MEDIUM ONION, COARSELY CHOPPED

4 CLOVES GARLIC, CHOPPED

10 BUTTON MUSHROOMS, FINELY CHOPPED

FRESHLY GROUND PEPPER

2 CUPS SPINACH, COARSELY CHOPPED

9 OUNCES FETA CHEESE, CRUMBLED

1 PINT GRAPE OR CHERRY TOMATOES, HALVED

Preheat oven to 475°F. Using a tablespoon, scoop out zucchini centers to form "canoes," leaving a 1/4-inch border. Roughly chop centers; set aside. Arrange zucchini, cut sides down, on a rimmed baking sheet; bake 15 minutes. Remove from oven. Meanwhile, heat oil in a large skillet over medium. Add onion and 1/2 teaspoon pepper; cook, stirring, until soft, 3 to 5 minutes. Add chopped zucchini, mushrooms and garlic, and cook, stirring, until most of the liquid has evaporated, about 8 minutes. Remove from heat; let cool slightly. Fold in feta, spinach and tomatoes. Turn hollowed-out zucchini cut sides up, fill with vegetable-feta mixture, and bake until top is lightly browned, about 20 minutes. Lift zucchini from baking sheet with a wide spatula, and serve. Serves 4.

The Practice: Like this recipe, yoga is a state of recognizing that we are all one. Stuffing the zucchini with these amazing delights creates an awareness of connection. All these ingredients coming together to create an exciting new explosion of flavor reminds us, if we work together, we can create a new world order. Yoga is about having a new experience by using all the things we know, mixing it up, and creating something new. Once we are in a space of our oneness, we activate the divine creation within us.

Mind Awareness Meditative Instruction: In a seated or standing position, connect your mind and thoughts to one body part. As you think about the body part, breathe and become aware of how it feels. Send thoughts of healing and awakening energy to that particular body part and repeat until you have blessed each part. The meditation can also be done by taking a moment to contract or squeeze each body part, beginning with the hands and moving up the arms and repeating until the body is alive and awake. Empowering thought and mantras, along with breath, will enhance the meditative practice.

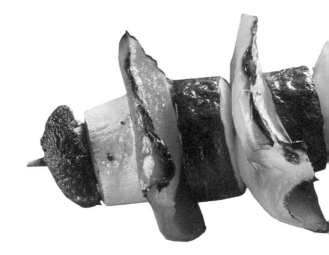

The Lotus Kitchen

Vegetable Kebabs

2 ZUCCHINI, CUT INTO 2 CHUNKS

2 YELLOW SQUASH, CUT INTO 2 CHUNKS

8 OUNCES FRESH MUSHROOMS, CLEANED

2 RED AND GREEN BELL PEPPERS CUT INTO 2 CHUNKS

2 MEDIUM RED ONIONS, CUT INTO WEDGES

2 EARS SWEET CORN, CUT INTO 2 CHUNKS

16 WHOLE CHERRY TOMATOES

8 OUNCES TERIYAKI SAUCE

Wash vegetables except mushrooms. Brush mushrooms clean. Cut vegetables to size according to recipe. Thread vegetables onto skewers. (If using wood skewers make sure you soak them.) Place on grill over medium-hot heat. Grill 20 minutes or until tender, turning frequently. Serves 8.

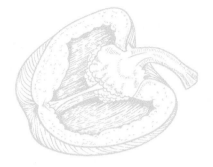

The Practice: In yoga, the Funnel mudra is when one has the hand lifted in the air with an open heart, representing a funnel. This funnel is meant to pour the goodness of life into one's heart, with arms wide open, and receptive and willing to receive the blessings of the earth. Each vegetable used in these kebabs is full of the goodness of the earth. With each bite be aware of the blessing Mother Earth is placing upon you. Always be willing to accept the goodness that mindful eating brings.

The Funnel Mudra: In a seated or standing position connect your mind and thought to one body part. Raise both arms up in the air, open to receive your blessing. As you think about the body part, breathe and become aware of how it feels. Send thoughts of healing and awakening energy to that particular body part and repeat until you have blessed each part.

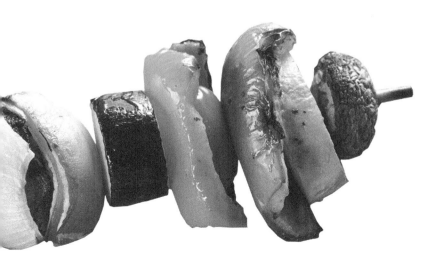

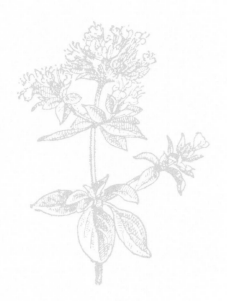

Cajun Grilled Eggplant

6 SMALL (BABY) EGGPLANTS
2 TABLESPOONS PAPRIKA
2 TABLESPOONS CAYENNE PEPPER
1 TABLESPOON PEPPER
6 CLOVES OF GARLIC, MINCED
3 TABLESPOONS ONION FLAKES
2 TABLESPOONS DRIED OREGANO
SALT

Wash the eggplants and slice them in half. Mix all of the seasoning ingredients together with a mortar and pestle until powdery.

Rub all over the eggplant on both sides and leave for 1-2 hours. Heat grill until hot. Spread some oil over the eggplant fillets and place on the grill, flesh side down. Cook for 5 minutes. Turn over and cook until done. Serves 4.

The Practice: In the yoga practice, there is a breathing known as "Ujjayi Breath" or Whisper Breathing. This practice is designed to internally heat the body. If done throughout the yoga practice, this becomes one's personal heating unit or grill.

The Ujjayi Breath Instruction: Ujjayi is a diaphragmatic breath, which first fills the lower belly, rises to the lower rib cage then moves into the upper chest and throat. Breathing is done completely through the nose, creating a whisper sound or an ocean tone, hence the name "whisper breathing." With a slightly constricted voice box the passage of air moves through which creates a rushing sound, internally heating the body.

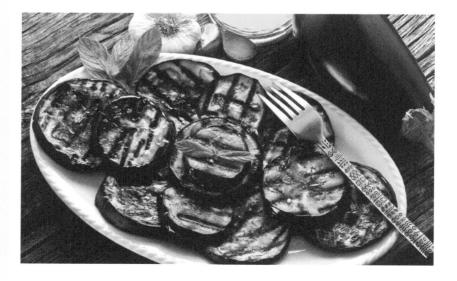

Noni's Zucchini Lasagna

3 POUNDS ZUCCHINI, SCRUBBED
5 CUPS TOMATO SAUCE
2 POUNDS RICOTTA CHEESE OR
   CASHEW CHEESE (RECIPE FOLLOWS)
4 CUPS SPINACH, FINELY CHOPPED
2 TABLESPOONS PARSLEY, CHOPPED
1/2 TEASPOON EACH DRIED
   OREGANO, BASIL AND NUTMEG

SALT AND PEPPER TO TASTE
1 CUP GRATED PARMESAN CHEESE OR
   NUTRITIONAL YEAST
1 POUND MOZZARELLA CHEESE,
   COARSELY GRATED OR DAIYA
   VEGAN "CHEESE"

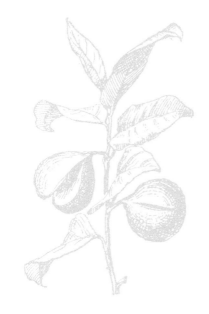

Slice zucchini into long slices. Cook in boiling water just until limp, about 5 minutes. Drain on paper towels. Combine ricotta, spinach, parsley, seasoning and half of the Parmesan cheese in a bowl. Set aside. In a 9×13 pan, spoon a thin layer of tomato sauce. Arrange layer of zucchini over this. Spoon half of the reserved ricotta mixture on top of the zucchini. Sprinkle with half the mozzarella cheese. Arrange the rest of the zucchini over this, layer more tomato sauce and top with remaining ricotta mixture. Top with remaining mozzarella and Parmesan. Bake in a 350°F oven for about 1 hour or until top is brown. Let stand 10 minutes before cutting.

Cashew Cheese

1 1/2 CUPS RAW CASHEWS
1 LEMON, JUICE AND ZEST
3 TABLESPOONS NUTRITIONAL YEAST
1/2 TEASPOON SEA SALT, TO TASTE

COMBINATION OF FRESH HERBS
   — OREGANO, THYME, BASIL,
   ROSEMARY

Place the cashews in a bowl and add several cups of filtered water. Let them soak overnight. This will soften the cashews and make them creamier and easier to process. Drain the cashews and place them in the bowl of a food processor. Add the lemon juice, zest, salt, nutritional yeast, and process for about a minute. In order to make the cheese as creamy as possible, stop the food processor occasionally and scrape down the sides. Continue processing until the mixture becomes creamy and starts to hold together, almost with the same consistency as ricotta cheese. Add in your combination of fresh herbs. Makes about 2 cups.

The Practice: Children love lasagna, and it's time to revisit the child within. Take time to remember how it felt to be a child. Play more, laugh more, sing more; observe the children in your life and allow them to help you reconnect with the inner child.

Child's Pose (Balasana) Instruction: On the mat kneel with knees hip-distance apart. Sit your hips back onto the heels of your feet, hinge forward from the hips and lower the head to the mat in front of your knees. Reach the arms behind you toward the feet and surrender like a child. Remember what it felt like to be free as a child, expressing love and joy, and one with ease and grace.

Wasabi Veggie Packet in Hawaiian Ti Leaf

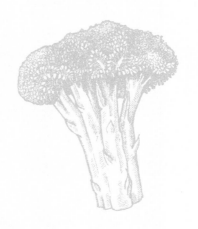

1 1/2 POUNDS ROUGHLY CHOPPED SEASONAL VEGETABLES — BROCCOLI, EGGPLANT, CARROTS, SUMMER OR FALL SQUASHES, PEAS, CAULIFLOWER, ASPARAGUS, BRUSSELS SPROUTS. ANY VEGETABLE WORKS; WE LIKE TO USE AN ASSORTMENT OF THE COLORS OF THE RAINBOW.

1/2 CUP OLIVE OIL

3 TABLESPOONS TERIYAKI SAUCE

1/2 TEASPOON WASABI PASTE

1 INCH PEELED GINGER, MINCED

3 CLOVES GARLIC, MINCED

SALT AND PEPPER TO TASTE

1 RED BELL PEPPER, JULIENNED

1 SMALL WHITE ONION, CHOPPED

4 HAWAIIAN TI LEAVES OR 4 BANANA LEAVES OR FOIL

Preheat grill for medium-high heat. Chop the veggies evenly in large pieces. Place veggies in a large bowl. In small bowl combine oil, teriyaki sauce, wasabi, garlic and ginger. Season to taste. Toss the vegetables with the wasabi mixture evenly to coat.

Place one ti leaf on a cutting board. Place vegetable mixture in the center of the leaf and wrap tightly like a package. Bottom to top and then the sides fold in and tie with kitchen twine or a thinly cut strip of an extra ti leaf. (You can also wrap the whole package in foil.) Repeat with the next 3 ti leaves. Place on the grill and cook for 15 minutes, flip them and cook 15 minutes longer. Unwrap your ti leaves and you will have a special Lau-Lau plate on which to enjoy your vegetables.

The Practice: The ti leaf is a sacred tea leaf that has been used in Hawaiian cooking for generations. This leaf is the perfect tool to hold the food in place while cooking on an open flame or grill. Like the ti leaf, the yoga mat helps us to stay in place during the practice. The yoga mat is our own personal ti leaf. Extended Child's Pose is the perfect way to connect with your yoga mat as if you were wrapped up in a ti leaf of yoga love.

Extended Child's Pose Instruction: On the mat kneel with knees hip-distance apart. Sit your hips back onto the heels of your feet, hinge forward from the hips and lower the head to the mat in front of your knees. Reach the arms long in front of the body, extending the reach as far as you can — reaching, spreading the fingers wide and sitting deep between your knees.

Roasted Veggie Wraps

5 CUPS ASSORTED VEGETABLES, ROUGHLY CHOPPED
6 CLOVES GARLIC, CHOPPED
3 TABLESPOONS OLIVE OIL
3 TABLESPOONS BALSAMIC VINEGAR
SALT AND PEPPER TO TASTE
1 CUP TOMATO SALSA
1 CUP HUMMUS
1 POUND WHOLE WHEAT LAVASH BREAD

Place vegetables and garlic on a sheet pan and coat with olive oil and balsamic vinegar. Season to taste and roast in a 400°F oven for 20 minutes until tender. Let cool and then toss with the salsa and hummus. Place one sheet of lavash bread horizontal on a cutting board. Place 1/6 of the veggies on the bottom half of the bread. Start at the end closest to you and roll away from you. When complete cut in half or in thirds and place on a plate or wrap in foil. Makes 12 halves that will serve 8 to 10.

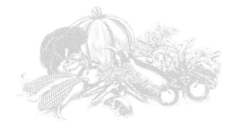

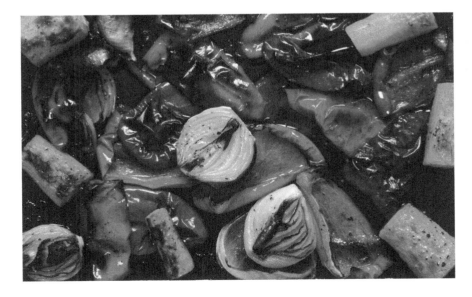

The Practice: Like a roasted veggie wrap that elevates the positive sensation of taste, yoga is a practice to help release fear. The Vanishing Fear Practice is done to activate positive energy within, and release the negative fear that we can hold on to.

The Vanishing Fear Instruction: Sit in a comfortable sitting position with the spine straight. Place the arms out parallel to the floor with the hands like a fist, except the thumb that is pointing outward. Inhale and bring the thumbs to the shoulders, exhale and straighten the arms back to the side. It's done as fast as you can to stimulate the pituitary gland. While performing this pose create a mantra or affirmation that helps to release your fear, for example: "All fear is released from my life!"

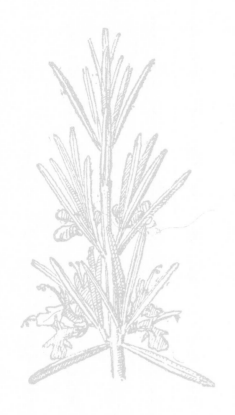

Rosemary Skewered Tempeh

1/4 CUP FINELY CHOPPED GARLIC, MASHED TO A PASTE WITH
   1 TEASPOON COARSE SALT
3 TABLESPOONS MINCED FRESH ROSEMARY LEAVES PLUS SPRIGS FOR
   GARNISH
4 TABLESPOONS OLIVE OIL PLUS OIL FOR BRUSHING TEMPEH
2 POUNDS TEMPEH

In a large bowl stir together garlic, minced rosemary, and 3 tablespoons oil. Add tempeh and marinate, covered and chilled, at least 4 hours or overnight. Thread the tempeh with the rosemary skewer. Grill 3 to 4 minutes on each side, or until just cooked through.

The Practice: Tempeh is a soy product from Indonesia that requires fermentation. Fermentation is the process of chemicals converting carbohydrates to alcohol, or through heat transforming one thing to another. Yoga is the ultimate fermentation of the mind, body and spirit. The chemical transition is happening throughout the practice. Our energy is shifting, there are endorphins being released and we begin to feel better. Like the alcohol, it can create a dizzy euphoric feeling. When feeling uneasy remember the child pose. Rest and be still. It is still yoga.

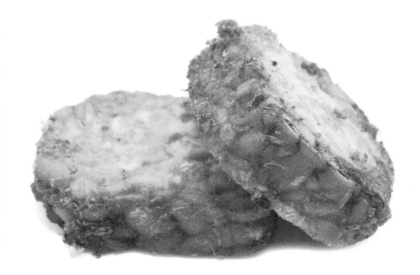

The Lotus Kitchen

Shiitake Mushroom and Vegetable Skewers

1 LARGE LEMON

1 TABLESPOON OLIVE OIL

1/2 CUP DIJON MUSTARD

1/2 CUP PINOT GRIGIO OR ANY LIGHT VINEGAR

4 CLOVES GARLIC, FINELY CHOPPED

1-2 INCHES OF FRESH GINGER, PEELED AND FINELY CHOPPED

1/2 TEASPOON FRESHLY GROUND PEPPER

1/2 TEASPOON CRUSHED RED PEPPER

1 POUND SHIITAKE MUSHROOMS

1 LARGE RED ONION, SQUARED

16 MUSHROOMS

2 YELLOW OR GREEN BELL PEPPERS

8 CHERRY TOMATOES

In a small bowl juice the lemon and add 2 teaspoons lemon zest. Combine the oil, mustard, vinegar, garlic, ginger, ground black pepper and crushed red pepper. Cut onion in half and each half into quarters. Cut the bell pepper in half and de-seed it and cut into 16 pieces. Clean the mushrooms. Dividing equally and then alternating them, thread the mushroom with all the veggies ending with the cherry tomatoes on 8 12-inch skewers. (Don't forget if using wood they need to be soaked in water for about 1 hour.) Brush with half the marinating mixture and let sit in the refrigerator for 1 hour. Prepare your grill. When it is ready, brush the skewers with half the remaining marinade. Grill the skewers about 5 inches from the heat for 5 minutes. Turn over and grill about 5 more minutes. Serve at once. Serves 8.

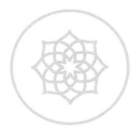

The Practice: Skewers are the process of bringing different delights together on a stick and grilling them to perfection. The skewer in yoga is called the Sutra. A Sutra literally means a thread or line that holds things together. Throughout the practice the Sutra is your intention. The intention is what keeps you in alignment with self and on the right track. As you make this dish, be aware of the intention. Before you practice, create your Sutra, set your intention for the practice. Although the Eagle Pose requires twisting, we must find the Sutra, the common thread that runs from the root chakra to the crown chakra.

Eagle Pose (Garudasana) Instruction: Stand tall on the mat and extend both arms to reach to the sides of the room. Bring both arms in front of you until the right elbow is under the left, continuing to wrap the arms around each other, joining the arms in the Namaste position. Sit back into Chair pose; place the right knee over the left knee and balance on one leg. After five breaths release the pose and contemplate the energy of the body. Repeat on the other side.

Grilled Bell Peppers Smothered in Black Bean Sauce

2 (15-OUNCE) CANS BLACK BEANS

1 TABLESPOON PEANUT OIL PLUS MORE FOR BRUSHING PEPPERS

1 RED ONION, CHOPPED

2 RED PEPPERS

2 YELLOW PEPPERS

2 GREEN PEPPERS

2 ORANGE PEPPERS

3 GARLIC CLOVES, CHOPPED

1 JALAPEÑO PEPPER, MINCED

1 CUP VEGETABLE STOCK

FRESH CILANTRO, COARSELY CHOPPED

The Practice: India is the second largest producer of the peanut, producing 6.25 metric tons a year. Peanut oil is used for cooking because of its mild flavor and a relatively high smoke point, which means it can withstand a high measure of heat. Yoga is the practice of allowing us to see how much heat we can tolerate or challenged we can be with the stand. During your practice, imagine yourself anointed with peanut oil. When you want to break from a pose, know that you can stand still for one more breath. Be strong like the peanut oil.

Tree Pose with Funnel Mudra (Vrksasana) Instruction: Root firmly the standing leg into the mat and spread the toes widely. Raise the opposite leg to the ankle, right below the knee or above the knee. Reach arms in the air and expand the arms to create a V shape representing a funnel that pours Divine blessing directly into the heart.

In saucepan heat peanut oil and sauté onions, jalapeño pepper and garlic for 5 minutes. Add peppers and cook until softened, stirring constantly. Add the black beans and stock and stir over medium heat until it thickens and sauce reduces about half. Puree with an immersion blender. We like to leave it a little chunky. Cover while preparing the peppers. Slice the peppers in half and remove the seeds and white pith. Prepare the grill low to medium heat. These can be done on the stovetop grill or broiler as well. Brush peppers well with oil and sprinkle with salt and pepper. Grill or broil until cooked through, about five minutes per side. If you made the sauce ahead reheat. Spoon sauce over peppers and garnish with fresh cilantro. Serves 6.

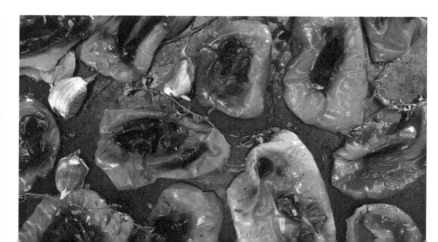

Grilled Eggplant Steaks with Pineapple Salsa

1/4 CUP OLIVE OIL
JUICE OF 1 LIME
JUICE OF 1 LEMON
2 LARGE EGGPLANTS, SLICED 1/2 TO 3/4 INCH THICK

Prepare the grill. Mix the oil and lemons and lime in a small bowl and brush over the eggplant generously. Grill the eggplant steaks 5 inches over the heat for about 6 minutes per side until they are firm to the touch. Remove from grill and serve immediately with a generous amount of salsa. Serves 6.

Pineapple Salsa

1 MEDIUM-SIZED PINEAPPLE
JUICE OF 2-3 LIMES
JUICE OF 1 LEMON
SALT, TO TASTE
1/4 CUP FRESH GINGER, VERY FINELY SLIVERED
1 WHITE ONION, CUT INTO THIN SLIVERS
1 TO 2 SMALL RED CHILIES, DRIED OR FRESH, STEMMED, SEEDED AND CUT INTO
   VERY THIN SLIVERS
1/2 CUP CILANTRO, COARSELY CUT

Peel pineapple, remove the "eyes," then core. Slice and cut into thin, matchstick slivers. Add lime and lemon juices, sugar, salt, ginger and onion. Taste for intensity of flavor; add additional sugar and/or salt if needed. Add chili slivers very sparingly, tasting until you reach the degree you prefer. (Caution: The heat will intensify as the salsa stands.) Just before serving, stir in cilantro. Best served within an hour or two of mixing.

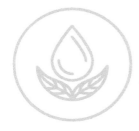

The Practice: Pineapple is one of the sweetest fruits the universe has created for our treat. Although yoga can be challenging, we must find the sweetest moments the practice can offer. Today find the joy. Find the joy in cooking, eating, and yoga. Ask the Universe, "Show me the joy." It will come. Have faith.

Chair Pose (Utkatasana) Instruction: Stand tall on your mat and spread the legs hip-distance apart. Anchor your feet by spreading your toes. Sit your hips back as though you are sitting in a chair. Reach your arms long toward the sky, lengthening the torso diagonally while spreading the hands. Look toward the hands and contemplate awareness of the body.

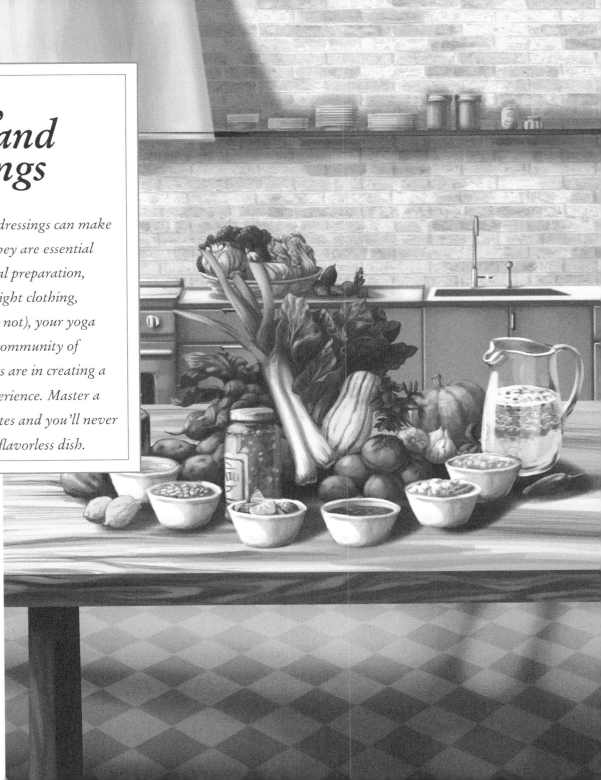

Sauces, Salsas and Dressings

Sauces, salsas and dressings can make or break a dish. They are essential components to meal preparation, just as mood, the right clothing, the right music (or not), your yoga teacher and your community of fellow practitioners are in creating a fulfilling yoga experience. Master a few of your favorites and you'll never know a boring or flavorless dish.

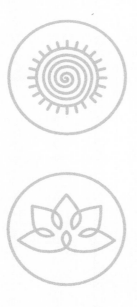

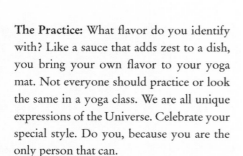

Asian Marinade

6 GARLIC CLOVES, FINELY CHOPPED
2 INCHES GINGER, FINELY CHOPPED
I BUNCH MINT LEAVES, CHOPPED
I BUNCH CILANTRO, CHOPPED
I BUNCH BASIL, CHOPPED
3 GREEN ONIONS, SLICED
2 SERRANO CHILIES, FINELY CHOPPED
I/2 CUP OLIVE OIL
I/2 CUP RICE WINE VINEGAR
JUICE OF 4 LIMES AND ZEST
I/4 CUP SOY SAUCE
I/4 CUP HONEY
I TABLESPOON CHILI SAUCE

In a large bowl whisk all ingredients together. Let sit for at least 1 hour or overnight. Makes 2 cups, enough for 12 cups of vegetables.

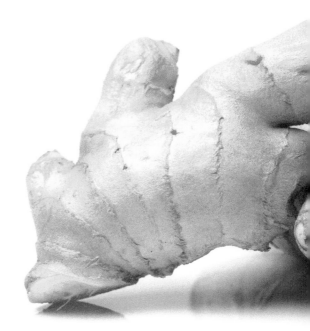

The Practice: What flavor do you identify with? Like a sauce that adds zest to a dish, you bring your own flavor to your yoga mat. Not everyone should practice or look the same in a yoga class. We are all unique expressions of the Universe. Celebrate your special style. Do you, because you are the only person that can.

The Lotus Kitchen

Pineapple Mango and Ginger Salsa

1 MEDIUM-SIZED PINEAPPLE, DICED

2 MANGOS, DICED

JUICE OF 2-3 LIMES

JUICE OF 1 LEMON

SALT TO TASTE

1/4 CUP FRESH GINGER, VERY FINELY SLIVERED

1 RED ONION, CUT INTO THIN SLIVERS

1 TO 2 SMALL JALAPEÑOS, VERY THINLY SLICED

1/2 CUP CILANTRO, COARSELY CUT

Gently toss together. Taste for the intensity of flavors. The heat intensifies the longer it stands. Let stand for 20 minutes to 1 hour for the flavors to gel. Makes 3 cups.

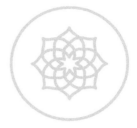

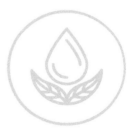

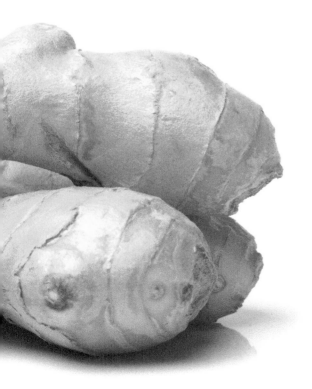

The Practice: Like the hot and spicy taste and feeling of salsa, Long Back Chair Pose or Bear Pose awakens the hot and sexy feeling of the body temple. While eating the salsa, be mindful of the energy you feel within the stomach and the groin area. Be aware of what is awakening within you.

Long Back Chair Pose or Bear Pose Instruction: From chair pose open legs wide and straddle the mat. Lower the chest between the knees and stretch the arms to the front of the room.

Heirloom Tomato Salsa

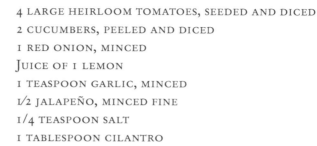

4 LARGE HEIRLOOM TOMATOES, SEEDED AND DICED
2 CUCUMBERS, PEELED AND DICED
1 RED ONION, MINCED
JUICE OF 1 LEMON
1 TEASPOON GARLIC, MINCED
1/2 JALAPEÑO, MINCED FINE
1/4 TEASPOON SALT
1 TABLESPOON CILANTRO

In a bowl combine all ingredients except the cilantro and chill, covered, until ready to serve. Before serving, toss in the cilantro. Makes 3 cups.

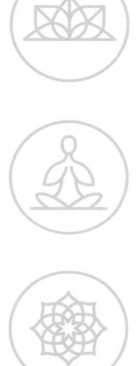

The Practice: The yoga accessory is nice, but it is not the yoga practice itself. Yoga mats, straps, and blocks help to bring the practice alive, more comfortable. Sauce is like the yoga accessory; it brings the food alive. Choose the sauce that will help to bring your dish to life, and remember you don't always have to use the same sauce.

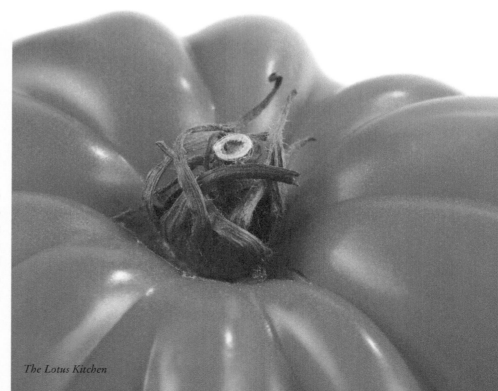

The Lotus Kitchen

Vegan Caesar Salad Dressing

No need for a raw egg or anchovy paste in this spin on a classic dressing. It embodies the salty sweet citrusy balance of the texture and great taste of the original.

1 FRESH FIG OR 3 DRIED FIGS
3 TABLESPOONS DIJON MUSTARD
8 KALAMATA OLIVES
JUICE OF 1 LEMON
¾ CUP BALSAMIC VINEGAR
UP TO 3 CLOVES OF GARLIC TO TASTE
2 TABLESPOONS DRIED THYME
2 CUPS OLIVE OIL

In the bowl of a food processor fitted with a steel blade pulse together the fig, mustard and kalamata olives to make a paste. Add the lemon, balsamic vinegar, garlic and thyme. Pulse on low and add the olive oil in a steady stream until well mixed. Makes 4 cups.

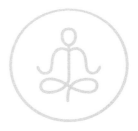

The Practice: Just like we can select a sauce or dressing, we also get to choose our yoga instructor. The instructor leads the class in his or her special way, adding to the practice a distinct flavoring. Find the instructor you like, and partake of the dish that speaks to you.

Music can help or distract your practice. Like any sauce or dressing we must choose wisely; we want to enhance the experience. Music is just a flavoring for the food of yoga. The music is not a box that we allow ourselves to be trapped in. You can do yoga to any music that suits you. Your music can be briny like the Caesar dressing, or it can be mild like sweet mango chutney. It's your choice.

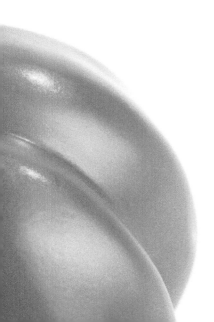

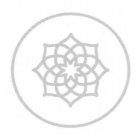

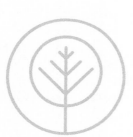

Lemon Shallot Dressing

In a jar mix the following:

Juice of 4 lemons
1 cup olive oil
1 shallot, minced
3 cloves garlic, minced
Salt (to taste)
Crushed red pepper (to taste)

Shake vigorously and serve. Makes about 20 servings.

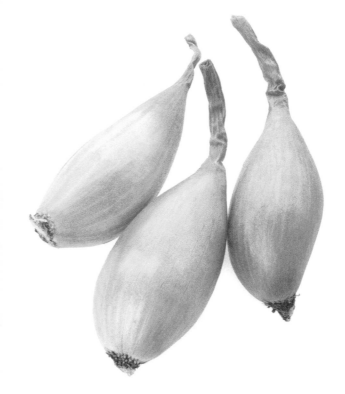

The Practice: Finding the right yoga studio is like finding the right salad dressing; you must try a few and taste the offering. Get out and find a space that speaks to you. Like the moment you know that a salad dressing tastes good, you will have the same internal feeling. You will intuitively know when you have found your yoga home.

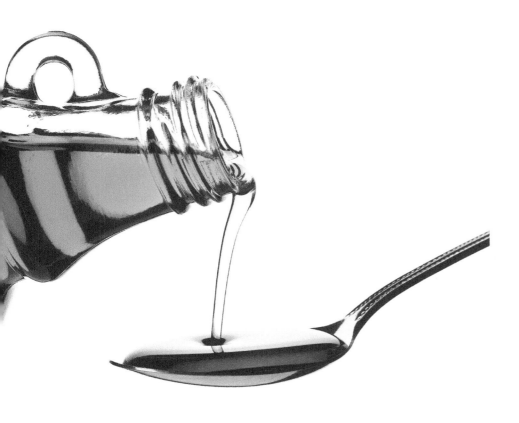

Maple, Garlic and Balsamic Dressing

2 CLOVES GARLIC, FINELY CHOPPED
2 TABLESPOONS DIJON MUSTARD
1 TABLESPOON MAPLE SYRUP
6 TABLESPOONS BALSAMIC VINEGAR
1 CUP OLIVE OIL
FRESH GROUND PEPPER

Whisk ingredients together. Makes about 20 servings.

The Practice: Food and yoga are each journeys; we must be willing to experience the unique joy they offer individually and collectively. Not every yoga practice or recipe will be alike. We are all different so we must take the journey to realize what we like, and what we don't. Life would be boring if we all liked the same sauce, or food, or yoga styles. Let the journey go, find you, and enjoy life while you are doing it.

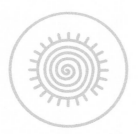

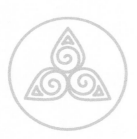

Pesto

5 LARGE GARLIC CLOVES
1 CUP PINE NUTS (WALNUTS WORK AS WELL)
5 CUPS PACKED FRESH BASIL
1 CUP FRESH PARSLEY
1 CUP FRESH PARMIGIANO-REGGIANO CHEESE, COARSELY GRATED
1 1/2 CUPS OLIVE OIL

In a blender or food processor mix garlic, nuts, basil, parsley and cheese and process until finely chopped. With motor running add oil, mixing until incorporated. Makes 2 cups.

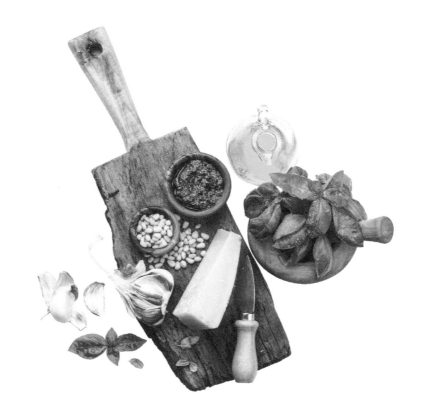

The Practice: Have you ever played the pesto mystery game? Take a bite of pesto and try to guess what's in it. Fun and tricky, that clever little pesto. The word "pesto" means to pound or crush into a flavorful paste. There are many ways to make pesto using a wide variety of ingredients. Just by being present and aware of the food you are eating, you will know all the ingredients in each and every dish. The practice is to know your own authority. Like yoga there is no wrong or right, just ask yourself and trust. Mindful eating is the same practice. Ask the body what it needs and expect an answer. Like guessing the ingredients in pesto, the revelations will be made known to you.

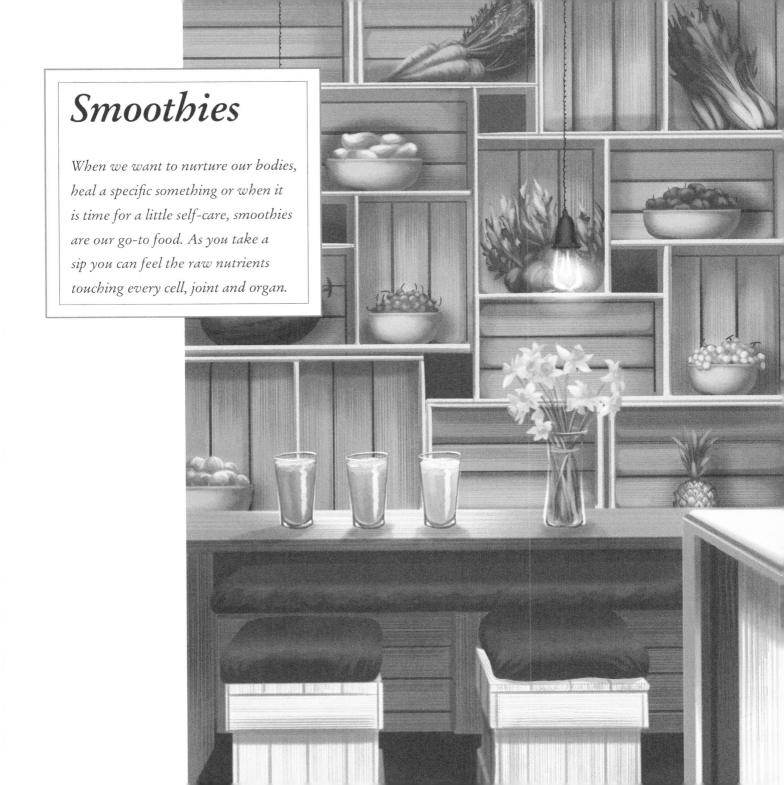

Smoothies

When we want to nurture our bodies, heal a specific something or when it is time for a little self-care, smoothies are our go-to food. As you take a sip you can feel the raw nutrients touching every cell, joint and organ.

Green Lotus

2 RIPE FROZEN BANANAS
1 CUP FROZEN COLLARD GREENS
1 CUP FROZEN SPINACH
2 TABLESPOONS PEANUT BUTTER
4 CUPS ALMOND MILK
1 SCOOP OF VEGAN PROTEIN POWDER

Place in blender and pulse until smooth. Makes 2 smoothies.

The Practice: "108 Japa Mala" — A Mala is a string of beads used to count mantras in sets of 27, 56 or 108 repetitions. The bead provides a starting and ending for counting the repetitions. Mala beads are an ancient tool developed to keep the mind focused during the practice of meditation. In yoga the Mala is used during the beginning or closing meditations allowing ample time for the practice. During the making of the smoothie use an affirmative mantra to bless the drink. "This smoothie is filled with goodness" is a simple chant while preparing your drink.

108 Spinal Mobility Instruction: Standing tall on your mat, begin by placing your hands on the hips with feet hip-distance apart. Inhale to begin, then squeeze the shoulder blades and expand your chest forward on the exhale. Inhale back to natural spine; exhale by closing your shoulders toward the midline of the body, then repeat 108 times while repeating your chant or mantra. Be mindful of any spinal injuries or discomfort you might feel. Listen to your body. At first do as many protractions/retractions of the scapulae that is right for you and then work your way up to 108. There is no hurry to get there, just the practice and the healing journey.

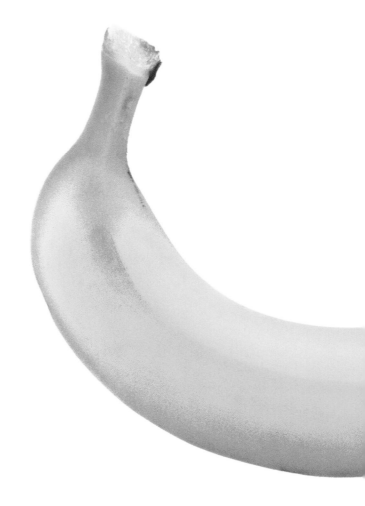

Sweet Green Smoothie

This is the smoothie of all smoothies. It's best if made and immediately consumed but can hold up if you prepare in the morning and place in a cooler bag for a later meal. Each ingredient has its own healing components but the real star in this smoothie is the coconut oil. It can boost thyroid function, helping to increase metabolism, energy and endurance. Coconut oil, an antioxidant, can also help our bodies resist bacteria and virus. It also keeps you full and satisfied, making this ideal for a breakfast or lunch to prepare for an extended yoga class.

2 BANANAS

2 CUPS PINEAPPLE

2 CUPS KALE

I CUP SPINACH

2 CUPS ALMOND MILK

I INCH GINGER, CHOPPED

2 TABLESPOONS COCONUT OIL

I-2 CUPS ICE

Place in blender and pulse until smooth. Makes 2 smoothies.

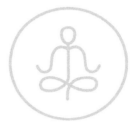

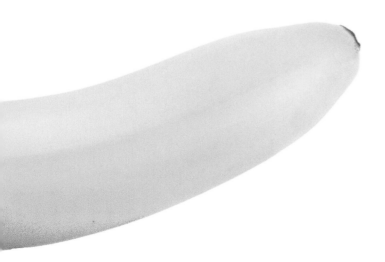

The Practice: The Goddess Pose Using Pranayama Energy. Yoga has been used through the centuries to harness sexual energy. By practicing specific poses you can actually improve your own sex life. The Goddess Pose connects you to your sexual energy and, like a Kegel, it strengthens the pelvic floor. Lay on the floor. Bring the soles of your feet together as close to your buttocks as possible. Place your right hand on your belly and your left hand over your heart. Close your eyes and inhale deeply, blowing up your belly like a balloon. Exhale and squeeze the breath out through your mouth, contracting your abs at the end. Repeat several times. Then squeeze the muscles you use to stop urinating, hold for 1 or 2 counts, then release; repeat 10 times.

Mama's Piña Colada

2 CUPS PINEAPPLE
2 TABLESPOONS COCONUT OIL
I TEASPOON VANILLA
2 CUPS ALMOND MILK

Using a blender add all of the ingredients except the ice and blend until well mixed. Then add the ice and blend again until smooth. Makes 2 shakes and can easily be doubled.

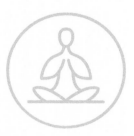

The Practice: Thich Nhat Hanh, spiritual leader and guru, says that when one is washing the dishes, one should wash the dishes. In other words, be present with whatever you are doing. One of the meditation principles is to be present. While preparing this simple smoothie recipe, be present. How does the pineapple smell? Perhaps enjoy a nibble of pineapple while blending the drink, being aware of the flavor and texture as it dances on your palate.

Upward-Facing Dog Pose (Urdvha Svanasana) Instruction: Lay flat on the mat, stomach down in prone position. Place hands flat on the floor under the arms. Press the hands onto the floor and straighten the arms. Drop the shoulders from the ears and lift the hips off the floor, keeping the legs straight and the feet flat and connected to the mat.

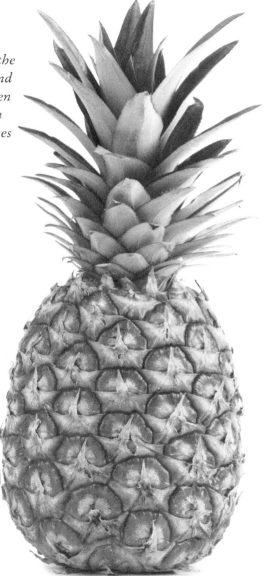

Sweets

Dessert is the ribbon on the gift that is your meal. A treat to be savored, it's also a mindful expression of love. Prepare these with love, serve with love and you'll taste the love with each delicious bite.

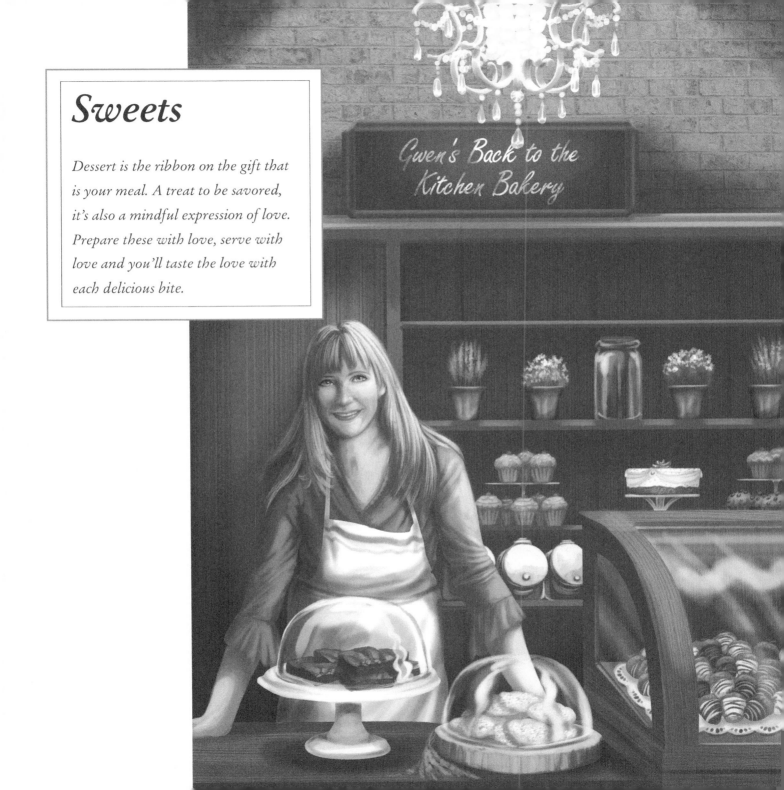

Strawberries Dipped in Heavenly 60% Chocolate

Chocolate makes us happy. It releases the same endorphins and serotonins to the brain as when we fall in love. And eating an ounce of dark chocolate a day can help reduce bad cholesterol and lower blood pressure. Chocolate is a loving gesture, to those we love and to self too.

8 OUNCES 60% CACAO BITTERSWEET CHOCOLATE CHIPS
1 POUND STRAWBERRIES WITH STEM, WASHED AND DRIED COMPLETELY
3 OUNCES WHITE CHOCOLATE (TO GARNISH)

Place chocolate in heatproof pan. Fill a medium saucepan with a couple inches of water and bring to a boil over medium heat. Turn off the heat; place the pan of chocolate over the water to melt. Stir until smooth.

Once the chocolate is melted and smooth, remove from heat. Line a sheet pan with parchment or waxed paper. Holding the strawberry by the stem, dip the fruit into the dark chocolate, lift and twist slightly, letting any excess chocolate fall back into the pan. Set strawberries on the parchment paper. Repeat with the rest of the strawberries. Melt the white chocolate the same way and with a fork drizzle over half of the strawberries for a lovely presentation. Serves 4 to 6.

The Practice: Laughter Yoga combines laughter with yogic breathing (Pranayama). Laughter is simulated as a body exercise in a group, activating our childlike qualities. Like a great dessert that stimulates endorphins and joy, Laughter Yoga allows the joy to flow during exercise. Today, choose a yoga pose and just begin to laugh, and laugh hard. Allow the vibration of laughter to elevate you to another level of being.

Namaste Laughter: A partner is needed. Put your hands together in front of your chest with palms facing the heart and laugh as you bow to one another. No words need to be spoken. Acknowledge the light within each other.

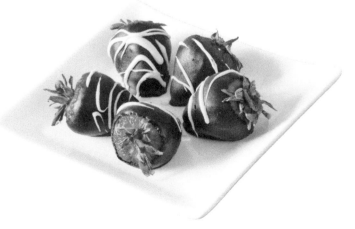

The Lotus Kitchen

Agape Agave Brownies

2 CUPS WHOLE WHEAT PASTRY FLOUR OR GLUTEN-FREE FLOUR

1 CUP AGAVE NECTAR

1 CUP UNSWEETENED COCOA POWDER

2 CUPS 60% CACAO BITTERSWEET CHOCOLATE BAKING CHIPS

1 TEASPOON BAKING POWDER

1 TEASPOON SALT

1/2 CUP WATER

1/2 CUP COCONUT OIL

1 TEASPOON VANILLA EXTRACT

COCONUT FLAKES FOR GARNISH

Preheat the oven to 350°F. In a large bowl stir together the flour, sugar, cocoa powder, baking powder and salt. Pour in water, coconut oil, chocolate chips and vanilla; mix until well blended. Spread evenly in a 9x13-inch baking pan. Bake for 25 to 30 minutes in the preheated oven, until the top is no longer shiny. Let cool for at least 10 minutes before cutting into squares. Makes 20 squares.

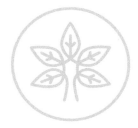

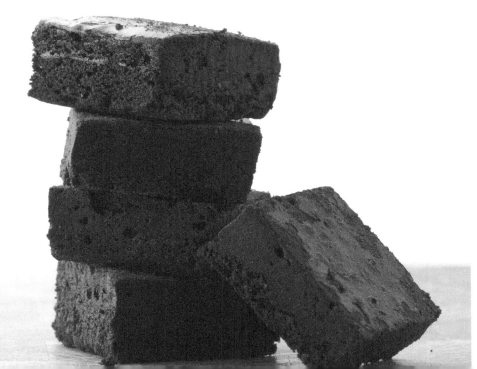

The Practice: The Smiling Meditation is the practice of sitting in a peaceful and comfortable position and just smiling to the deepest part of your soul. Imagine the smile flooding every part of your body. This energy-shifting practice has been known to heal the body temple and change one's perception on life. Like a delicious agave brownie, smiling is the dessert for the soul. While eating this treat, just smile and feel the overwhelming joy as it is being delivered to your body temple.

The Smiling Meditation Instruction: Find a space to sit comfortably. Relax and close your eyes and simply smile deeply into your soul. Imagine the smile traveling through your body, a light and happy journey. Be aware of your feelings. Take as much time as you need. The smiling meditation is healing for every part of the body.

Coconut Macaroons

This cookie is a gracious addition to a dessert table, or stands proudly on its own. It only contains three ingredients and they all contain many health benefits. Brown rice syrup raises blood sugar but doesn't make you crash the way other sweeteners do and many enthusiasts say it's the only sweetener they'll use. It can be a bit sticky to work with but the end result is divine and so worth the effort.

2 CUPS SHREDDED DRY COCONUT
3 TABLESPOONS VANILLA ALMOND MILK
2/3 CUP BROWN RICE SYRUP

Preheat oven to 350°F. In a bowl combine almond milk and coconut. Let sit for about 1 hour. Add the rice syrup and mix with your hands. Using a small ice cream scoop, fill tightly and place on a wax-paper-lined baking sheet. Repeat until you have 24 little scoops. Bake for 15 minutes. Allow the macaroons to cool completely before removing from the baking sheet. Makes 2 dozen.

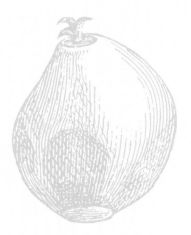

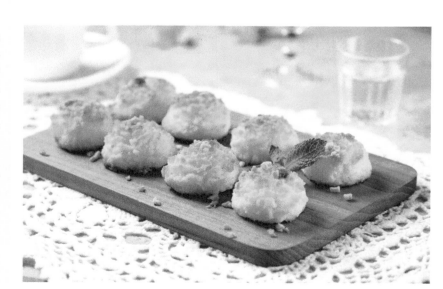

The Practice: Yoga was created by people who wanted to mimic an animal or amendment object to become one with what they saw. It's the practice of becoming one with everything. Like desserts, yoga can be a fun and delightful experience. Try the yoga game to help you find your joy.

Name the Pose — Yoga Game Instruction: Yoga Game: Name My Pose? Like desserts, yoga can be shared with family and friends. The yoga game is simple and joyous. One person strikes a pose and everyone gets to guess what it is. Have fun with your desserts and have fun with your yoga.

Apple Tarte Tatin

4 OUNCES AGAVE NECTAR
3 TABLESPOONS BUTTER
1 TEASPOON CINNAMON
3 LARGE GRANNY SMITH APPLES, PEELED, CORED AND THINLY SLICED
1 SHEET PUFF PASTRY, THAWED

Preheat oven to 350°F. Grease the bottom of a 9-inch cake pan with butter. Cover the bottom with agave. Sprinkle the cinnamon evenly over the agave. Arrange the apple slices over the cinnamon, fanning them out from the center and overlapping the slices. Lay the sheet of puff pastry over the pan and cut to fit. Tuck down evenly over the apples. Cook for 40 minutes or until puff pastry is golden brown. Remove from oven and allow to rest on wire rack for 10 minutes before inverting onto serving plate. Make sure your serving plate is tightly placed over top of the tarte tatin before flipping it over. Be careful — the sauce is extremely hot and can burn you if you are not cautious. Let it drip for a couple minutes before removing pan. Serves 6.

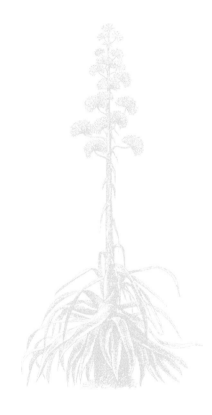

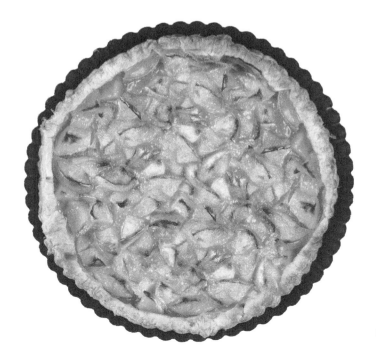

The Practice: Yoga Game — Yoga ABCs are a fun way for the kids to get moving. One person calls out the ABCs and the other participants make letters with their bodies. Apple Tarte Tatin is a rich dessert so to balance the delicious goodness, let's keep moving.

Lavender Sable Cookies

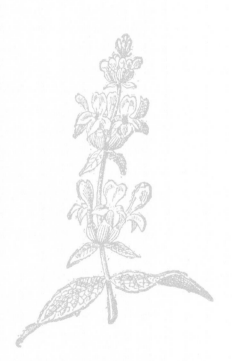

1 1/2 STICKS UNSALTED BUTTER, SOFTENED AT ROOM TEMPERATURE
3/4 CUP POWDERED SUGAR
1 EGG YOLK
PINCH OF SALT
1 TABLESPOON DRIED LAVENDER
ZEST FROM 1 LEMON
1 3/4 CUPS FLOUR
3 TABLESPOONS CORNSTARCH

Sift flour and cornstarch, set aside. With an electric mixer, beat butter on medium speed until smooth, add powdered sugar and beat until well blended. Beat in the egg yolk, followed by salt, dried lavender and lemon zest. Add the flour mixture and blend with a spatula. Mix gently until flour is incorporated. Gather dough to form a ball, divide in half and wrap each piece in plastic wrap. Chill dough for 30 minutes in refrigerator. Form each piece of dough into a log that is about 1 to 1 1/4 inches in diameter. Wrap logs in plastic wrap and chill dough for at least 2 hours in refrigerator or leave overnight. When ready to bake, preheat oven to 300°F. Once the oven is ready, slice the log into 1/4-inch-thick pieces and place on a lined baking sheet with 1/2-inch intervals. Bake for 15 minutes or until the cookies are set but not brown. Transfer to wire rack and let cool completely. Makes 2 dozen.

The Practice: The Sweet Smell of Life. This practice is all about smelling the flavors the universe has in store for us. Lavender is a strong delightful fragrance. When was the last time you sat and smelled the flowers? Yoga is the pathway to a deeper awareness of all the senses. The practice is to take your yoga out into nature. Smell the flowers, smell the trees, practice outside with Mother Earth, and watch your yoga blossom.

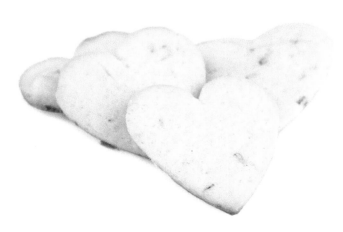

The Lotus Kitchen

Baked Pear, Cranberry and Apple

4 PEARS, CHOPPED
4 APPLES, CHOPPED
1 CUP DRIED CRANBERRIES
1/2 CUP AGAVE NECTAR
1/2 TEASPOON CINNAMON
1/2 TEASPOON CHINESE FIVE-SPICE

Topping
1 CUP QUICK COOKING OATMEAL
1 CUP CHOPPED NUTS

In a square glass pan toss together apples, pears, cranberry, agave and spices. In a bowl mix the oatmeal and nuts. Sprinkle over the fruit mixture and bake in a preheated 350°F oven for about 40 minutes until bubbly. Serves 6 to 8.

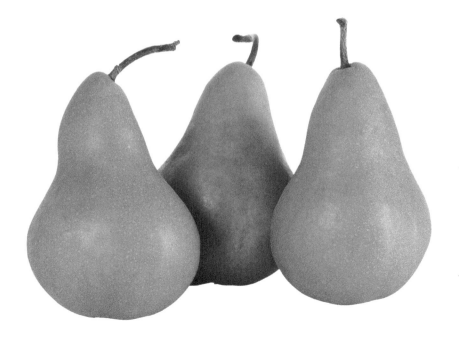

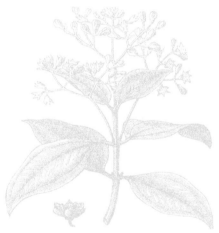

The Practice: Yoga Game — Swami Says. Swami Says is another yoga game that will bring joy for your family and friends. Like Simon Says, Swami will call out a pose but the participant can only move if they hear "Swami Says" first. Like the baked fruit treat, this yoga game will bring a smile to the faces of all who participate.

Raw Chocolate Bars

1/2 CUP COCONUT OIL
1/2 CUP CACAO POWDER
1/2 CUP BROWN RICE SYRUP
1 TEASPOON VANILLA EXTRACT
1/2 CUP CHOPPED HAZELNUTS

Beat liquid ingredients until super smooth. You can add more sweetener or more chocolate to suit your taste. Transfer mixture to separate bowl and stir in chopped hazelnuts. Spread on a plastic-wrap-lined plate or dish and place in freezer to cool. Break into pieces to serve. Serves 6 to 8.

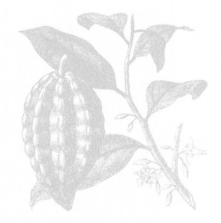

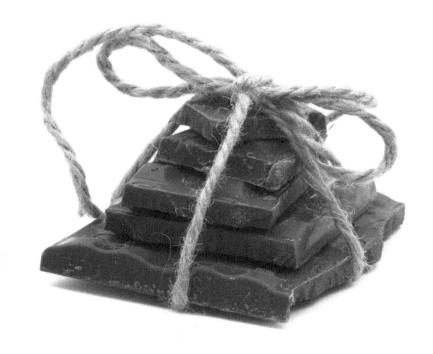

The Practice: Relax and do nothing but enjoy life. Take your chocolate bars and sit in a nice warm bath and contemplate how good life is. Allow the Joy to be activated. Yoga has two sides to the practice: the Yin and the Yang. The Yang is the Doing and the Yin is the allowing. Sometimes we need to stop doing, and just sit and allow. Yoga is about knowing when to move, and when to sit still.

Grandma Kay's Zucchini Bread

1 CUP GRAPESEED OR SUNFLOWER OIL

1 CUP BROWN SUGAR

3 EGGS

1 TABLESPOON PURE VANILLA EXTRACT

2 CUPS GRATED ZUCCHINI

3 CUPS FLOUR

1 TEASPOON CINNAMON

1 TEASPOON SALT

1 TEASPOON BAKING POWDER

1/2 TEASPOON BAKING SODA

1 CUP COARSELY CHOPPED WALNUTS

1 CUP RAISINS OR DRIED CRANBERRIES

Preheat the oven to 325°F. Oil 2 5x9-inch loaf pans. In a large bowl, combine the oil and brown sugar. Add the eggs, one at a time, beating after every addition. Stir in the vanilla and zucchini. In a smaller bowl, sift together flour, cinnamon, salt, baking powder and soda. Stir the dry ingredients into the oil and the egg mixture until just moistened. Fold in the raisins and walnuts. Spoon batter into the prepared loaf pans. Bake for about 1 hour, until a knife in the center comes out clean. Makes 2 loaves.

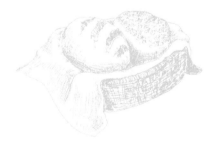

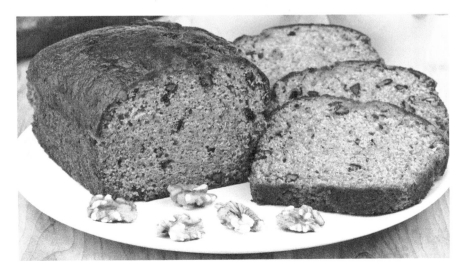

The Practice: Yogi Game — Yogi See, Yogi Do. Dessert time should be fun, and so can yoga. Yogi See, Yogi Do is a simple game of follow the leader. One person does a pose, and the other tries to copy the pose. Have fun, and enjoy the other person's creativity.

Zucchini Pie

8 CUPS ZUCCHINI, SLICED AND CUT IN HALF
1 CUP SUGAR
2/3 CUP LEMON JUICE
1 TABLESPOON LEMON ZEST
1 TABLESPOON CINNAMON

In a saucepan cook sliced zucchini, sugar, lemon juice, and cinnamon until zucchini is tender (about 10 minutes).

Crust:

4 CUPS FLOUR
2 CUPS SUGAR
1/2 TEASPOON SALT
1 1/2 CUPS BUTTER

Mix together the flour, sugar, salt, and butter until crumbly. Pat half crust mix into 9×13 pan. Bake 10 minutes at 375°F. Add 1/2 cup crust mix to hot cooked zucchini mix; cool. Pour over baked crust. Add 1 teaspoon cinnamon to remaining crust mix. Spread over zucchini filling. Bake at 375°F for 35 minutes; cool. Cut into squares.

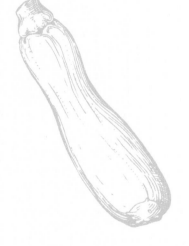

The Practice: When we think of pie, we often think of a singular slice of a pie. Yoga is about discovering your wholeness. Like a pie, each slice is essential to create the entire pie. See your mind as a part of the pie, see your body as another part of the pie, and your spirit as the final slice of your wholeness. You are a complete, whole pie of goodness. Today we celebrate your divine wholeness, and how complete you really are.

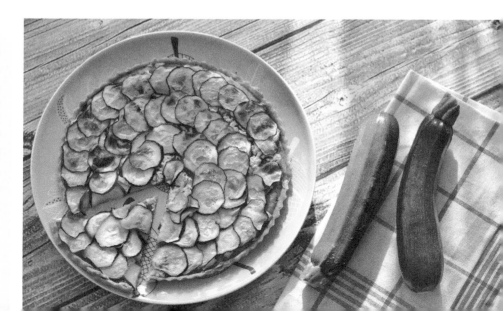

The Lotus Cookie

This delight was created for a crew on a film set and even the fiercest sweet tooth reveled in its flavor while marveling at its "good for you" status. It seemed fitting to name it after our beloved lotus, given its birth during the final days of writing this book.

4 CUPS ALMOND MEAL
1/2 TEASPOON SEA SALT
1/2 TEASPOON BAKING SODA
1 TEASPOON CINNAMON
3/4 CUP COCONUT OIL, MELTED
1/2 CUP MAPLE SYRUP
1 TABLESPOON VANILLA
1 CUP CHOPPED DARK CHOCOLATE OR 1 CUP DRIED CRANBERRIES
1/2 CUP CANDIED GINGER

Preheat the oven to 350°F. Mix the almond meal, salt, baking soda, and cinnamon. Stir in the coconut oil, maple syrup, and vanilla. Stir in the chopped chocolate (or cranberry) and ginger. Drop by rounded tablespoon onto ungreased baking sheets. For a variation, sprinkle a little sea salt before baking. Bake for 10–12 minutes on parchment-paper-lined cookie sheet until the edges are golden. Let them rest on the pan for 5-10 minutes to firm up before removing. Makes 3 dozen.

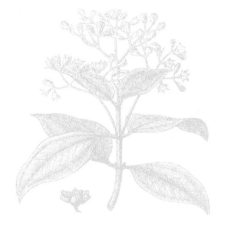

The final practice: Each yoga class ends with the practice of Namaste. The Lotus Kitchen Namaste is performed by placing your hands on your third eye and allowing your hands to drift to Anjali mudra in front of the heart chakra. Close the eyes and bow down to show deep respect for self, others and our practice.

The Namaste gesture represents the belief that there is a divine love within each of us, located in the heart chakra. Nama means bow, as means I and te means you. Namaste literally means "bow me you" or "I bow to you." When I am in a place of Peace and Love and you are in a place of Peace and Love we are one. The divine love in me bows to the divine love in you. Namaste.

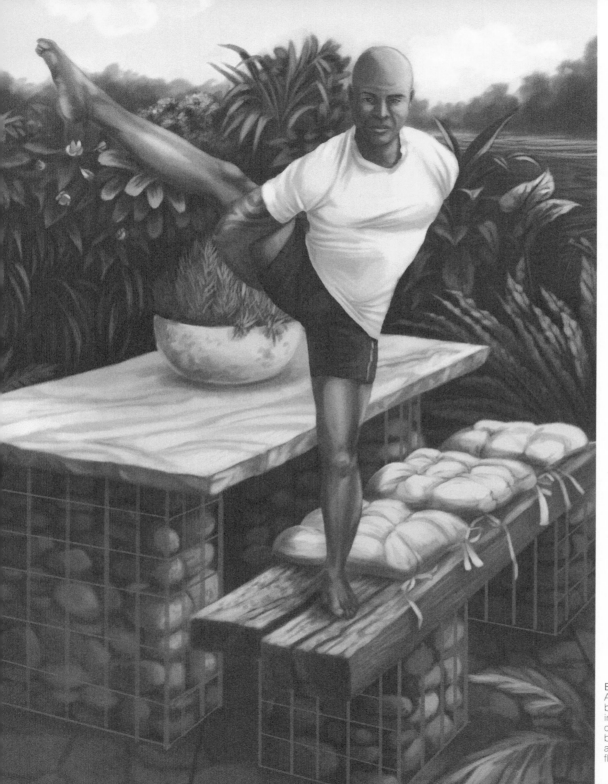

BIRD OF PARADISE
A challenging
balance pose that
incorporates hip
opening, core and
back strengthening,
and hamstring
flexibility.

From Gwen ~

In loving memory of Jim Sahin. Not only am I a better chef because of you, I am a better human being. To Rafet Sahin, Wendy Warren Lorenz, Serkin Sahin, Gil Barrios and the gang at Jimmy's Café Aldente — we baked pies, created ambiance, cooked together and became a family.

To my amazing clients at Back to the Kitchen Catering Company: Thank you for letting me play in your kitchen. And thank you to the best team ever: Rafet Sahin, Zelma Livingston, Louie Perez, Otto Krause, Romy Walthall, Rev. Rio Kelley. You shine your light so bright when you co-create with me. Thank you for always making me look good.

To Heather Marshall at Heather Sent: Thank you for allowing me to grow as a private chef and for becoming such a dear friend.

Katherine and Jack Kenneally — Mom is guiding me on this side of the veil and Dad on the other. You still make the perfect team.

Massive amounts of love to those who have enjoyed my food, practice and friendship: Linda Favila, Dawn Heinsbergen, Martin Mcilvenna, Lisa Jongewaard, Anastasia Morgan, Karen Young, Elizabeth Howell, Jonathan Howell, Lynn Kahn, Rick Kahn, Timothy Kenneally, Joy Graff, John Kenneally, Spencer Proffer, Steve Love, Dave DiGregorio, Matthew Kenneally, Kelly Kenneally.

And the young Kenneallys:
Claire, Ryan, Alex, Katherine,
April, Matilda, Katelyn.

Rev. Dr. Michael Beckwith,
Dr. Rickie Byers Beckwith, Rev.
Dr. Kathleen McNamara, Cory
Tyler, Rev. Dr. Coco Stewart,
April Rivera, Rev. Juliet Moret,
Dr. Lissa Sprinkles and everyone
at the Agape International
Spiritual Center — I am honored
to be a Licensed Spiritual
Practitioner and carry the Agape
Movement in all of my work
and play.

Skip Jennings: what a joy-
filled ride this has been. Thank
you for sharing the vision and
lifting me through the challenges
and the bliss in the ever
expanding Lotus Kitchen.

Judy Proffer: I love your
strength, beauty and grace. I
cannot begin to express the love

and gratitude for all you are and
all you have done for me.

To Emma Rose, my most
beautiful and loving yogi girl.
Thank you for choosing me to
be your mom. The gifts and
talents you bring to the planet
are immense. The Buddha says
"when you are open and ready
your teacher appears." Thank you
for teaching me about living life
to the fullest, creating fearlessly
and loving unconditionally.
Because of you I am forever a
grateful and willing student.

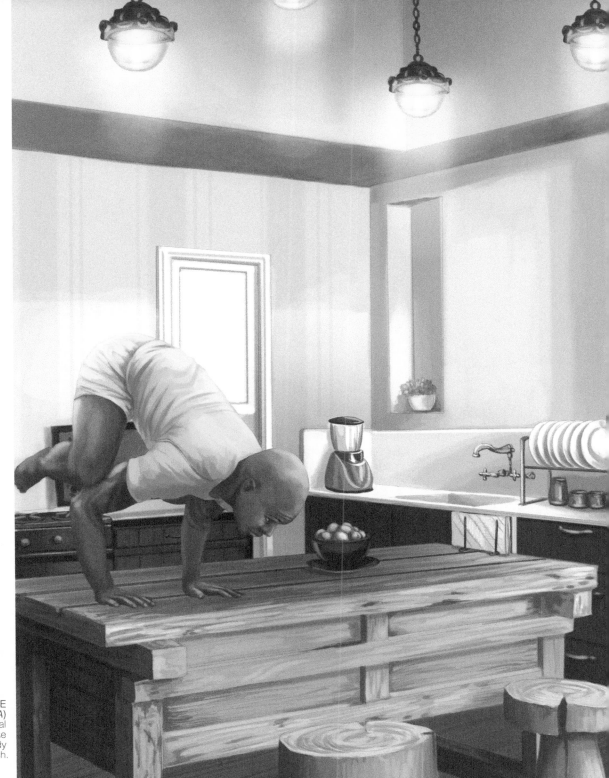

CROW POSE
(*BAKASANA*)
The quintessential
arm-balancing pose
for upper-body
strength.

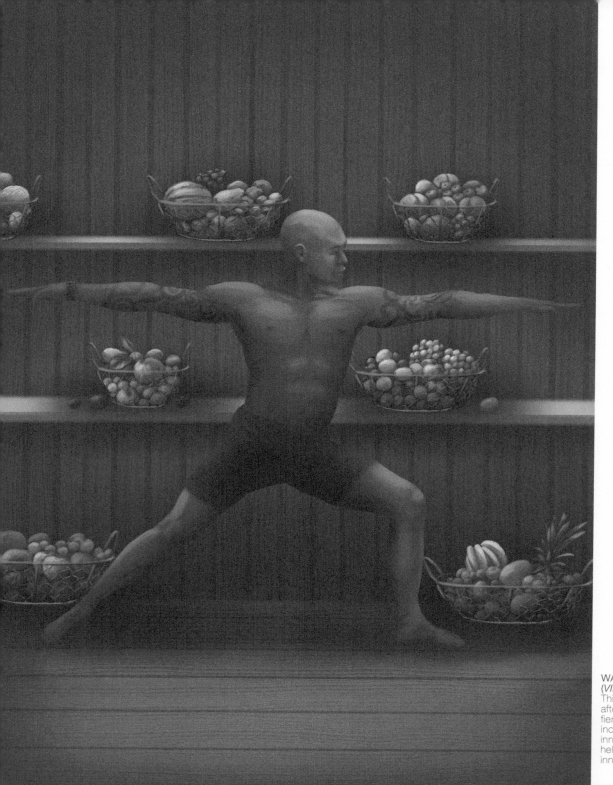

WARRIOR TWO (*VIRABHADRASANA II*)
This pose is named after Virabhadra, a fierce warrior and an incarnation of Shiva. An inner thigh opener that helps you tap into your inner Warrior Spirit.

From Skip ~

To my mother Rebecca Jennings, thank you for teaching me the value of healthy living. Before herbs, juicing and vegetarianism were trendy you introduced me to the path of holistic healing and for that I will always be grateful.

To my nephew Chaune "Chauncey" Jennings who inspired me to be a better man. You came to this planet with such a bright light and did what you needed to do. You made this world a better place. You continue to live on in my heart and I will never forget you.

To my sister and my guardian angel Beth, thank you for teaching me unconditional love. I am forever grateful for the time we shared.

This book is also dedicated to every yogi, vegetarian, vegan and light worker that says yes to a higher consciousness that heals this planet. Continue to live for the higher purpose and everything else will be given to you.

Thomas "T.J." Jennings, thanks for being my big brother. Love you!

Cynthia Jennings, you are the big sister that God blessed me with.

Thank you Chaia Jennings, my divine niece. I could not have asked for a greater blessing. I am so proud of you.

Bill Robertson, thank you for always being my Best Friend and sometimes editor.

To David "LaLa" Pavese, what a long and powerful

journey. You inspire me to ask the big questions. I thank God every day for your friendship.

Honey Labrador, your guidance and friendship have helped me to be the man I am today. Thank you!

Dr. Michael Bernard Beckwith, my life transformed when I stepped through the front doors of Agape. Thank you for seeing my light before I knew that it was on.

Gerrick Angel, there are times I ask and you always say "Yes." Thank you!

Tom Blumenthal, from client to friend, I will always be grateful to you.

Kat Stein of KNS Design — for the wonderful Malas I wear daily.

Gwen Kenneally, thank you for co-creating this work of art

known as The Lotus Kitchen. *What a journey. I remember telling you that I wanted to do a cookbook and by the end of the conversation, I knew I would write* The Lotus Kitchen *with you. Thank you for not letting me give up.*

To Judy Proffer and Huqua Press, thank you, thank you, and thank you. Dreams do come true. I am forever grateful. Your vision has taken our ideas from glory to greater glory!

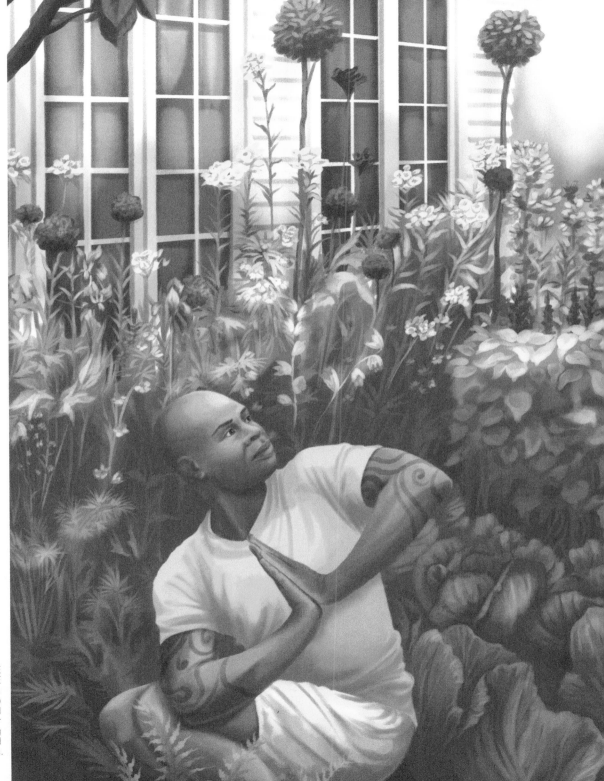

REVOLVE TOE
BALANCE POSE
(*PARIVRITTA
SAMATVAMASANA*)
This pose is designed
to challenge your
tbalance while training
your obliques and
core muscles.

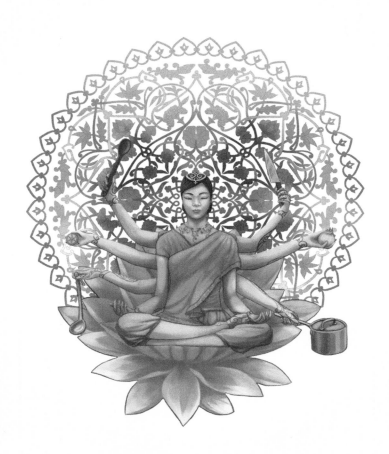

CPSIA information can be obtained
at www.ICGtesting.com
Printed in the USA
FSOW03n1642021015
11758FS

9 780990 696629